TRUE PREVENTION—

OPTIMUM HEALTH

Remember Galileo

*Ray,
Thank you for your presence and your friendship, your presence and friendship are blessings. Love,
Jeanine Joy*

Also by ♥ Jeanine Joy

"Trusting One's Emotional Guidance Builds Resilience",
Perspectives on Coping and Resilience. Ed. Venkat Pulla, Shane Warren,
and Andrew Shatté. Laxmi Nagar: Authors Press, 2013. 254-279

TRUE PREVENTION—
OPTIMUM HEALTH

Remember Galileo

♥ Jeanine Joy

Thrive More, Now

TRUE Prevention—Optimum Health:

Remember Galileo

A Thrive More, Now Book / May 2014

Published by
Thrive More, Now
Charlotte, North Carolina

All rights reserved
Copyright © 2014 Jeanine Joy

All rights reserved, including the right to reproduce this book or portions thereof in any form whatsoever. For information address: Thrive More Now publishing, Rights Department, P.O. Box 6888, Concord NC 28078

For information about special discounts for bulk purchases or speaking engagements, please contact Thrive More, Now.

**Edited by
Courtney Broderick**

**Cover Art:
Original art by Rosario Rizzo adapted by Jeanine Joy**

ISBN-13:

978-0615992464

9780615992464

ISBN-10:

0615992463

Dedication:

For all those who are asking and open to receiving information to help them thrive more, now.

With Love,

♥ Jeanine Joy

Contents

Contents

Contents 2
Chapter 1: Oh the Places We Will Go 1
Chapter 2: Cardiovascular Disease (CVD) 7
    "Risk Factors" 10
Chapter 3: Smoking 13
    Solutions 15
        Smokeless Tobacco and e-cigarettes 18
Chapter 4: Physical Activity 21
    Judgment and Stress 23
    Make Play OK™ Campaigns 26
Chapter 5: Weight Management 31
    Adverse Weight Judgments 33
Chapter 6: Nutrition 37
Chapter 7: Depression 41
Chapter 8: Bits and Pieces 45
    Addictions 46
    Type II Diabetes 51
    Cognition 53
    Colds and Flu 56
    Pain 57
    Occupation Related: Nurses 58
    Posttraumatic Growth and Resilience 60
Chapter 9: Perception 61
Chapter 10: Intro to Emotional Guidance 73
Chapter 11: Emotional Guidance Sensory Feedback System (EGS) ... 87
Chapter 12: Filtered Consciousness 107
Chapter 13: Beliefs, Expectations, Emotional Stance, and Focus 121
Chapter 14: Coherent Thought 131
Chapter 15: Happiness Defined 139
Chapter 16: Chronic Stress 145

    Being Positive or Positive Thinking 148

    Mindset and Emergencies...156

Chapter 17: Processes (How to Think Positive)...159

    Follow Your Guidance 161

    Shift Your Focus 164

    Positive Affirmations...168

    Think Positive..169

    Setting Intentions..171

    Forgiving 172

    Nature..173

    Exercise 174

    See the Potential in Others and in Self...................................174

    Meditation 176

    Go General...178

    General to specific 179

    Appreciation (not gratitude) 181

    Consider your Resources..183

    End Self-criticism...184

    Refute 187

    Use Role Models...188

    Stop Catastrophizing 189

    Use Big Picture Perspective to Prevent Arguments 189

    Breathe 190

    Handling Difficult Times... 191

Chapter 18: Permission to Self 195

Chapter 19: A Global Solution 207

Acknowledgments.. 211

Disclaimer...212

Send Me Your Stories 213

Feel Inspired to Help? 214

Are you a researcher? 215

Programs, Retreats, and Cruises 216

Bibliography 217

Chapter 1: Oh the Places We Will Go

Congratulations!
Today is your day.
You're off to Great Places!
You're off and away!
Dr. Seuss

My goal for TRUE Prevention—Optimum Health: Remember Galileo is to help humanity see the big picture of what makes humans thrive and provide practical how-to processes that work. I began asking, "What makes humans thrive?" twenty years ago. Once I found the answer, it was an epiphany for me to realize that different people wanted their knowledge in different flavors. Some wanted it to be purely scientific while others insisted new information be consistent their religious worldview[1].

As a result, I began asking another question, "How can I help as many people as possible with the information I have?" The answer was to create bridges from commonly accepted ideas to the more beneficial information, and just as an ice cream parlor offers chocolate, vanilla, and strawberry, I wanted to be able to explain what I'd found in the "flavors" to reach a larger number of people—so we all understand. I began building bridges from common beliefs about health, relationships, success, and well-being in three flavors: scientific, religious, and spiritual. Each has its own bridge—each one stands on its own merits.

Many nonfiction books can be read in pieces, reading only the chapters that are of interest. This is not that type of book. A tremendous amount of new information is provided. The prevention strategies build on information provided in preceding chapters. **The reader will gain the greatest benefit by reading this book in the order it is presented.** This book explains the scientific bridges from what we think we know to a less complex perspective supported by new scientific findings. I am writing separate books for the religious and spiritual bridges.

In order to prevent illness, we must understand what causes wellness. Illnesses, as the researchers and physicians have discovered, manifest themselves in different ways in each individual. This is the reason there is not one side effect for a medication; it can have different side effects with different people and no side effects with others. For the same reason, when we look at aspects of someone who is not well and notice others parts of their physicality that are not well, we cannot truly say those other aspects are the cause. They may very well be, and often are, symptoms of the illness we are examining.

In the first section of TRUE Prevention, I will provide a basis of understanding that highlights the fact that the "risk-factors" wellness programs most frequently address are actually symptoms, not risk factors. Then I will drill deeper into the individual "risk-factors," demonstrating that each of them shares a common root in the majority of the cases. Once the common root is established, I will further simplify the concept to the place where true wellness must be sought.

In recent years, many researchers, physicians, and others have made suggestions that seek to address the root, but those suggestions did not reach the deeper root. The same inconsistency of results was found in these suggestions; they worked for some people, but not for others. After I establish my premise, I will provide some processes that heal the deeper root problem and lead to greater wellness.

Along the way, I will make some big suggestions. My work has led me to see aspects of education that slow humanity's progress to a better world. One of my reviewers remarked that by referring to "humanity" I was separating myself from others. I appreciate knowing my intent could be misconstrued, so I will explain why I use it. Each of us has myriad labels applied to us throughout our lives, some even before we breathe our first breath. If I refer to changes using only language that states "we" or "our," it could easily be interpreted to mean I am referring only to those labels that are attached to me, such as American. My work will fundamentally change the entire world for the better in every critical area: health, relationships, success, and well-being. I intend it to benefit everyone who wants improvement in any of those areas. I want to benefit everyone because I feel a deep and profound connection with others.

Why me? How did I come up with these answers?

Scientists view problems they want to solve through different lenses. We all do. Some speak of genetics. Unfortunately, I seldom see the new field of epigenetics, an area where significant discoveries have been made in recent years, considered by the old school geneticists. Others view the world through an evolutionary lens. I understand it—new knowledge in one area can turn an education in another field on its head. The plethora of information coming out on a daily basis is mind-boggling.

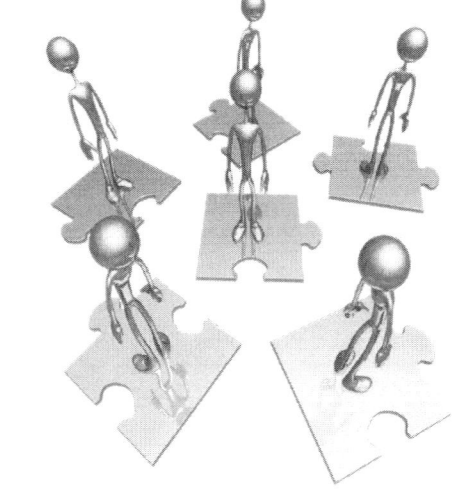

Separate branches of science study human thriving[2], but the pieces were not assembled into a whole. Research in one branch indicates they observed something, but did not understand what caused the outcome, prompting a call for more research to understand it better. The answer is not something that field of science can answer—it was something already answered by another branch.

Science has become so specialized that they sometimes miss the forest for the trees.

We spend years and enormous amounts of money training masses of people to see the world the same way, to accept the same ideas that their predecessors had—often accepting old, unproven premises as factual. Because I was not indoctrinated into the scientific mindset, I was uniquely suited to see the big picture. Most of the questions scientists ask are very specific, such as:

- What happens neurologically when someone does this or feels this way?
- What happens to the body's biochemistry when this happens?
- Why does someone develop (a certain type of) cancer?
- Are blueberries good for our body?
- Does this drug have a beneficial effect on this illness?

For the most part, a question like mine is considered so broad and general as to be unanswerable. Because I had not been indoctrinated into the mindset that believed this, I did know this in the beginning. The question pulsated within me and kept my attention for more than a decade. There is a saying, "Be careful what you ask for, you just might get it." This is true about my journey.

My research was conducted in my spare time until 2010—a hobby that occupied much of my non-working hours. To be clear, my research consists of finding, understanding, and compiling research others conduct. During working hours I was building a successful career in an unrelated field. As the big picture answer began forming, my after-hours research occupied increasing amounts of my time. Once I realized that what I can offer others by sharing this information is so much greater than any contribution I could make in my old career, it was no longer really a choice.

After the first decade of research, pieces of the puzzle were forming a pattern. My understanding of the answer grew rapidly. I shifted from looking everywhere to focusing on an idea that I initially expected to be a dead end—it was so radical and different from how I had always viewed the world. But the more I looked, the more evidence of its validity I found. The world began making more sense. The reason other premises have so many exceptions became clear to me. The root cause of undesirable things–illness, crime, addictions, and more were all related! One solution is **the solution.** They all share a common root cause.

When it all made sense, when the puzzle was complete, I founded Happiness 1st Institute to share the solution with the world.

I greatly appreciate the countless researchers who contributed pieces of the puzzle. Without their work, the big picture would not be explicable in scientific terms—or provable.

It is from the big picture perspective that the wonderful potential reveals itself—where the way everything humanity struggles with today is interconnected.

My goal in TRUE Prevention is to establish a firm foundation—a foundation that allows humanity to move confidently forward in healthier, more loving, and peaceful ways. There are two obstacles in our path. One is what I have termed the Galileo Effect. I use Galileo because most educated individuals are aware that Galileo proposed a new idea that was accurate and provided a better understanding of our world but his findings met with criticism, ridicule, and worse. Most of humanity seems to believe this sort of reception is something that less educated individuals did—that the people of today are too intelligent and too educated to treat the truth with disdain. I used to believe this, too. Now, I can demonstrate that we have repeated the same behavior throughout history and that it continues today.

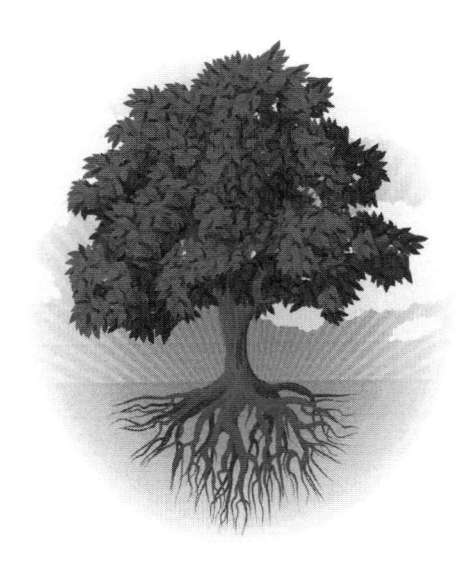

While beneficial progress always wins—eventually—a lot of suffering happens between awareness by some and adoption by the masses. My passion is fueled by my desire to avoid as much suffering as possible. Recognizing beneficial changes sooner is the easiest way to avoid unnecessary suffering. A methodology to help humanity increase their comfort level with new ideas faster is provided herein.

During my journey, many of my fundamental beliefs about life and the world were overturned. Much of the way I viewed the world, positions I staunchly defended not that many years ago, were based on false premises that do not serve humanity. The only perspective I can take that feels good about what I used to believe is appreciation that I now know more than I once did. If I were willing to take a different perspective, I could feel guilty for how I used to view the world, or dumb, or incompetent, or blind, or any number of perspectives that would not serve me or anyone else.

I do not insist that others agree with me. I do ask that this work is approached with an open mind—the opposite of the Galileo Effect.

In the second section of the book, I explore how most people view the world we share and introduce healthier perspectives that would enable each individual to thrive more. The third section includes processes that not only tell the reader what to do, but also a deep understanding of why the process works and the emotional states[3] at which it will be most beneficial. I close with a business case for organizations who wish to do their part to make Earth better for everyone by sharing this knowledge with their employees.

My work does not diminish the value of work that has gone before. The individual who contributed the least, contributed greatly. Individuals who worked for years to attempt to find cures that did not work contributed greatly. The quote with which I begin the next chapter is not intended to say anyone deliberately misled us. Each person does the best he or she can in any given moment. It is meant to point out that once we are convinced an idea is accurate, it becomes a truism regardless of the soundness of the idea. We like a solid platform. We tend to believe ideas others believe with unquestioning faith. We cling to those ideas even after overwhelming evidence that they are inaccurate exists. This is not a deliberate action on our part. It is not stubbornness or a lack of intelligence. In the chapter on filters, the reason for this is explained.

The second obstacle is that many foundational premises on which our societies are built must change in order to achieve the benefits of what science has shown is true. When many people understand the big picture, I am confident there will be a groundswell insisting on those changes. We want solutions to the social ills that plague our world and good health throughout life but many basic tenets accepted as truths today create the opposite. We are so close—we must move forward.

Chapter 1: Oh the Places We Will Go

Chapter 2: Cardiovascular Disease (CVD)

A lie's true power cannot be accurately measured by the number of people who believe its deception when it is told; it must be measured by the number of people who will go out after hearing it trying to convince others of its truth.

Dennis Sharpe

Cardiovascular Disease (CVD), or heart disease as it is commonly referred to, kills more people than any other cause. Worldwide, 17. 3 million die from heart disease every year[4]. Since the beginning of the Revolutionary War in the United States, 2,717,991 Americans have died or been wounded in a war[5]. It takes less than four years for that many Americans to die from heart disease. 2,200 Americans die from heart disease every day[6].

Half of these deaths may be preventable[7].

In June 2011, the National Prevention Council published the National Prevention Strategy, *America's Plan for Better Health and Wellness*. I was excited when I first saw the government was issuing a prevention strategy. I knew from my research how much good could be done to prevent unnecessary illness and death. Unfortunately, my excitement about the report was short-lived. In reality, the report did not address prevention of illness or disease. It addressed treating symptoms. The report included subtitles that indicated solid information that would actually help Americans thrive more such as "Empowered People" but the information provided in the sections with promising titles missed the mark—by miles.

> *Americans are not alone. A cursory review shows that Canada and the UK have similar prevention plans that overlook the potential for prevention that is known.*

First, the prevention plan addresses symptoms that increase the risk of developing heart disease. By the time someone has symptoms, they are already well on their way toward developing heart disease. You see, heart disease is not an isolated event that suddenly develops. It is near the end of a continuum that begins with unmanaged stress. The risk factors *America's Plan for Better Health and Wellness* addresses are well along the continuum. A more appropriate label would be "Symptom Management" or "Cost Management of Symptoms." **True prevention keeps an individual from being anywhere on the continuum leading to death from heart disease.**

America's Plan for Better Health and Wellness does not provide True Prevention. It does not educate Americans about the root cause of heart disease and almost every illness and social problem our country contends with. Everyone deserves access to this information—Americans and all the people of our world deserve to know how to thrive more.

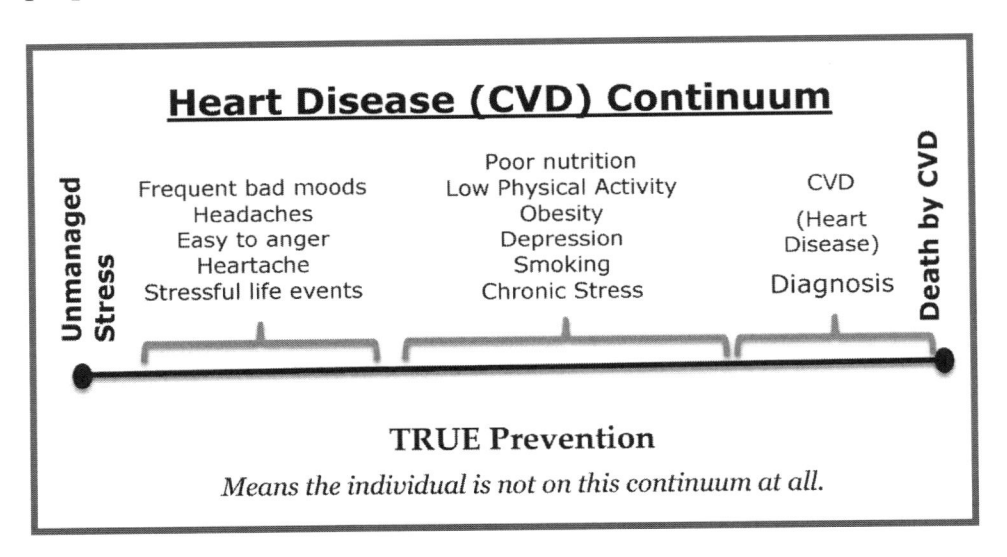

Heart Disease (CVD) Continuum

Unmanaged Stress →
- Frequent bad moods
- Headaches
- Easy to anger
- Heartache
- Stressful life events

→
- Poor nutrition
- Low Physical Activity
- Obesity
- Depression
- Smoking
- Chronic Stress

→
- CVD (Heart Disease)
- Diagnosis

→ **Death by CVD**

TRUE Prevention
Means the individual is not on this continuum at all.

Each "risk factor" for heart disease is, in fact, a symptom. Scientific evidence supporting this position for each symptom exists. Chapter 17 and 18 provide an array of processes individuals can utilize to prevent them from beginning the journey to heart disease.

Considerable evidence suggests the same strategies that support healthier bodies will positively affect every major social problem including crime, drug abuse, teen pregnancy, incomplete educations, high divorce rates, violence, and even war. Although I will not delve as deeply into these concepts as I do the health aspects, I will suggest the path. We have the knowledge and the means to reshape Earth in ways that support all life more fully.

Finally, the current rate of heart disease is a problem for everyone. Beyond the individual cost of shorter and less enjoyable lives, beyond the heartache of losing loved ones, everyone pays part of the economic cost as well. Annually, the direct cost of heart disease is estimated at $324 Billion[8]. The cost of lost productivity is estimated to be an additional $137 Billion[9]. If each person on Earth paid this cost proportionately, the amount due per person would be about $65 per year.

In 2012, a report in the Psychological Bulletin published by the American Psychological Association written by Harvard researchers stated the risk of developing heart disease could be reduced by 50% with increased positivity and optimism[10]. The significance of this report is tremendous for several reasons.

A lot of new information contradicts what I was taught in school. Science should be labeled, "What we believe is true today" or "What we think we know so far" to help us keep an open mind and not staunchly defend false information. Our teachers did the best they could with what they knew at the time. I am sure none of them deliberately taught false information.

First, it was not a single research study. It was a meta-analysis that reviewed 200 independent studies and reached conclusions based on the results of the other research. Second, the work was completed by researchers from a highly respected institution. Third, the study demonstrated that positivity and optimism is not only protective against heart disease, but that it increases healthy behaviors (adequate sleep, better nutritional choices, etc.). Increased healthy behaviors also have a preventative affect for other illnesses and diseases.

Another significant study reported that positivity and optimism increase life expectancy by 10. 7 years, and healthy life by 18 years.[11] In this study, debilitating end of life diseases not only came later in life, they came much closer to death. Many individuals do not want to extend their lives if the quality of their life is diminished during the additional years. This study highlighted that not only is life shorter for pessimistic individuals, they spent more years suffering from debilitating diseases than those who have the skills to maintain a positive outlook.

LUCKY OPTIMISTS?

Before we drill down to the negative impact of pessimism on our health, I want to be sure the pessimists have hope that they are not doomed to suffer long debilitating diseases and an early demise. In order to do this, a common but inaccurate belief about pessimism and optimism must be addressed. Otherwise, it just sounds like optimists are lucky.

If you are like me, you were raised to believe that pessimism and optimism are inborn traits, which individuals cannot change. This was once a predominant belief. Many of us learned it in school. Fortunately, science has shown this commonly held belief is false.

Since there is not a systematic notification to graduates that something they were taught in school is now known to be inaccurate, such beliefs tend to remain common long after the truth is known. Pessimists can do a lot to become more optimistic and gain the health and well-being benefits of a more positive outlook. New thought patterns can become so automatic that the old, pessimistic thoughts feel foreign.

A frequent objection arises from a belief that our personality is who we are. Later we will go into detail, but personality traits are a function of many things—most notably the current mood and habitual patterns of thought an individual practices. The real person, the part that does not change, is an improvement over the one who acts based on habitual patterns without having consciously decided to adopt them.

> *Optimism can be developed with skills anyone can use.*

The common fear that we might discover something bad about ourselves if we reflect too much is based on false premises. It requires a firmer foundation than is appropriate here.

The reason it was believed that people were either pessimistic or optimistic and could not change was because few people changed. Being optimistic or pessimistic is a habit—a habit of thought. Think about how difficult it can be to change your habits. Now imagine attempting to change a habit you did not recognize as being a habit in an areas where you had no training in how to modify. That is the only reason most people remained the same.

We live in a great time. We now know that pessimism is the result of habitual thoughts and have many techniques that successfully help individuals change undesired habits of thought. In fact, changing undesired habits of thought may be the easiest habit to change—when an individual understands how to do it. The reason is that there are immediate good-feeling results from intentional efforts to change negative patterns of thought. Unlike dieting or overcoming addictions, no pain is required for the gain.

"Risk Factors"

We must approach the epidemic of cardiovascular disease differently. Understanding the so-called risk factors are actually symptoms focuses attention on true prevention, not just symptom management. Symptom management is important for cost control and patient well-being in the short-term. The long-term goal of prevention is possible only by addressing the root cause.

Before we go further, I want to stress that most of the suggestions being made by physicians, wellness programs, and in *America's Plan for Better Health and Wellness* is helpful. The point is not whether those common suggestions are beneficial—most of them can be very beneficial. The critical point is that the "risk factors" are symptoms. To prevent heart disease, the underlying root cause must be addressed. This is actually great news. It is great news because every individual has the ability to take positive steps to benefit their health.

Six symptoms are commonly cited as risk factors for the development of heart disease. Most wellness programs exert most of their effort towards managing these symptoms. While the return on investment (ROI) from these efforts is cost effective, the results of addressing the root cause would provide a significantly higher return on investment (ROI) and provide significant benefits in other areas of concern, such as employee engagement and turnover. Also, it is important to note that positivity training not only reduces the risk of heart disease by 50%, it also leads to substantial improvements in the symptoms that are currently considered risk factors for heart disease.

Symptoms of the Heart Disease Continuum

So-called Risk Factors

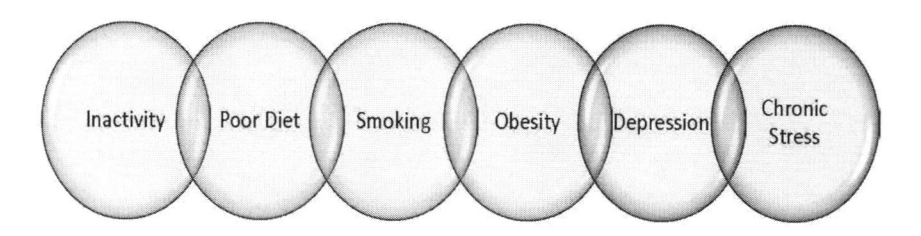

Inactivity | Poor Diet | Smoking | Obesity | Depression | Chronic Stress

The six symptoms that receive the most attention are low physical activity (inactivity), poor nutrition (diet), smoking, obesity, depression, and chronic stress. For example, in *America's Plan for Better Health and Wellness,* they encourage placing healthy food choices near the cash register to encourage better choices and making stairwells safer so people will choose to use them instead of the elevator. The report also states, "Clinicians can refer patients to community-based prevention resources such as programs for blood pressure and cholesterol control."

By the time someone's blood pressure or cholesterol is elevated, he already has a symptom of a disease that frequently results in heart failure. Powerful steps that reduce the risk of developing the symptoms are easier to accomplish than dieting, giving up smoking, or taking up an exercise program. The outcome of these steps increases the success of the actions currently recommended to combat these symptoms. A win-win for everyone involved—except the industries with a vested interest in maintaining an unhealthy populace.

Chapter 3: Smoking

Giving up smoking is the easiest thing in the world. I know because I've done it thousands of times.
Mark Twain

Most wellness programs focus efforts on providing education of the risks of the symptoms and attempting to coax employees to curb or cease unhealthy habits. Almost every smoker knows smoking is unhealthy—education is not the answer. In fact, when the education is done in a way that stigmatizes smokers or makes them feel guilty for their addiction, the programs often do more harm than good. The stigmatization and guilt reduce individual self-efficacy making becoming a non-smoker a more difficult task[12]. It also increases stress—which has significant health consequences.

The most successful non-smoking programs incorporate a behavioral change aspect in the program. There are a couple of ways to measure the success of a non-smoking program. One measure is how many people actually quit smoking, but the more important measure is how many quit and remain non-smokers on a long-term basis.

In this chapter, I will demonstrate that stress and anxiety hinder efforts to quit smoking. Stress management training will increase the success of efforts to encourage employees to quit smoking. Stress management training also improves the quality of life for the smoker and everyone he interacts with on a regular basis.

Just like the smoking cessation programs, most smoking prevention programs aimed at youths focus on educating them about the health risks of choosing to smoke. Children and young adults do not begin smoking because it feels good. The first puff is awful. The reason for beginning smoking in the first place can also be traced to poor stress management skills.

Many will point to peer-pressure as a cause. What is peer pressure? Is it not pressure to do something in a situation where going along with the group feels less stressful than not going along? We tend to train our children to please the people in their lives. Then, when they reach their teens and their attention shifts from pleasing parents to pleasing peers, we blame peer pressure. We train our children to listen to and follow what others want instead of listening to their own intuition and guidance. This creates all sorts of additional problems. Once a child is trained to please others, we have to worry about who they choose to hang around with—because we know their associates will influence their behavior and choices.

A child who decides for herself what is acceptable and not acceptable behavior—who places her own well-being above pleasing friends—will make better choices. If you've ever experienced negative peer pressure, I'm sure you recall not wanting to do something but going along due to the pressure from your peers. When the higher priority is following one's own guidance, that pressure simply does not exist. I have a daughter who followed the beat of her own drum in this regard. Several times during her teen years I noticed the sudden absence of a friend. At the root of this was always a decision by the friend to participate in behaviors my daughter wanted no part of. Not once was I aware the friend had begun engaging in unhealthy behaviors before my daughter chose to end the close relationship. If I had been attempting to control the situation by influencing the friends she was around, I would have been far behind where I wanted to be.

Teaching our children to please others and then sending them in the world really disables them. I can hear the resistance now—that not caring about what others want is selfish. This reveals one of the false assumptions that plague our society. The truth is that we want close relationships with others—we want to be kind and loving toward others. When we feel good, we are kind[13]. When we feel trapped, or forced to acquiesce to others' desires to please them, we do not feel good. When we feel emotionally worse, we are not as kind to others. The kindness of a positively focused happy person extends to strangers.

An individual trained to do what makes him happy will foster good relationships. They will be even better toward others because no resentment builds up over having to do something to keep another happy—they do the things they do to keep others happy because it supports their goals, which makes them happy. Many relationships decline because each person is expected to accomplish the impossible task of making the other happy. In their futile efforts, frustration and resentment builds. It is not possible to make someone happy unless and until that person has decided they want to be happy. Many people put things like being right ahead of their own happiness.

I have not traced the etymology of the viewpoint that making one's own happiness a priority is selfish. Adam Smith's quote, "It's not from the benevolence of the butcher, baker, or brewer that we expect our dinner, but from their regard for their own wellbeing" seems to indicate the Founding Fathers of the USA (or at least one of them) did not see taking care of one's own needs as selfish. The connection between the baker taking care of his own needs and the good of the community is clear.

Stress management training can effectively teach children to do what they believe is best for themselves and still feel good. It takes the need to please those who are not considering our own best interests out of the picture, reducing the pressure to go along with the crowd. Reducing the stress of such a situation increases the cognitive ability available to the individual, which allows him to use creative measures to exit the situation without compromise.

Sometimes the decision to smoke is an act of rebellion. Happy children do not rebel. Only someone under significant stress rebels against a rule that is in place for his or her own good. While many rules may be given this label by parents, in the case of smoking cigarettes, it is accurate to say that a rule not to smoke is in the child's best interest. How can you increase a teenager's chances of being happy and not rebellious? Help the child develop strong stress management skills.

SOLUTIONS

Why do smokers smoke when they know the health and social risks? Research shows smokers tend to be more anxious than non-smokers.[14] Skills that build resilient and calm thought processes lead to pro-health and pro-social outcomes and provide smokers with knowledge and skills to self-manage stress, anxiety, worry, and depression.

Stress management skills are so important to well-being in every area of life they really should be taught in school. The basics are easy enough for young children to grasp and successfully apply. Programs to teach stress management skills to children would greatly enhance efforts to prevent smoking.

Research shows that smokers are more anxious and have significantly higher rates of depression than non-smokers do.[15] Current major depression rates of 22% to 60% have been observed among smokers.[16] General population depression rates are estimated at 8.7%.[17] Depression reduces the successful quit rate (of those who attempt to quit) by 50%. It is linked with smoking cessation failure.[18] Depression also decreases the chances an individual will attempt to quit. Increasing self-efficacy has been shown to improve success for adults who wish to quit smoking.[19]

While I do not define happiness as the absence of stress, I see happiness and stress as two ends of the same continuum. Strong stress management skills cause changes in the way an individual perceives their ability to function in the world, easing worry about future events, and increasing confidence, which results in increased happiness. The following diagram shows the relationship between stress and happiness. The zones are discussed in Chapter 11.

Chapter 3: Smoking

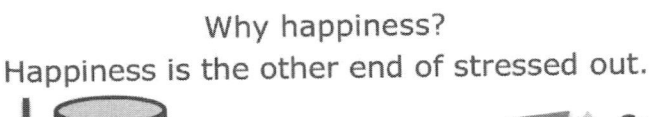

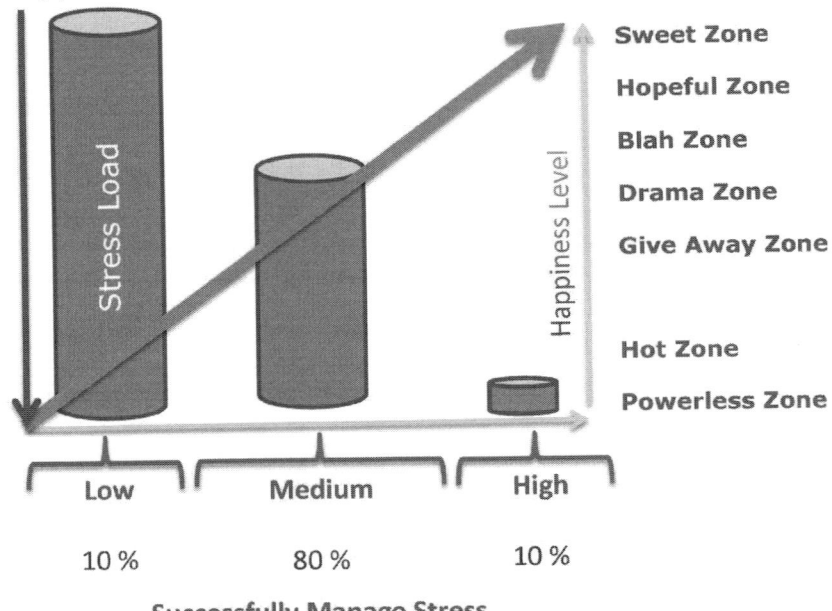

Why happiness?
Happiness is the other end of stressed out.

- Sweet Zone
- Hopeful Zone
- Blah Zone
- Drama Zone
- Give Away Zone
- Hot Zone
- Powerless Zone

Low — 10 %
Medium — 80 %
High — 10 %

Successfully Manage Stress

Once again, increasing stress management skills is a viable solution. Unhealthy habitual thought processes contribute significantly to the experience of anxiety and depression. Our schools attempt to teach what to think, but how to think and how to modify unhealthy thought processes is not taught to the general population. Habitual thoughts created a path of least resistance in your brain, which allows those thoughts to flow automatically. This can make changing your habits of thought seem difficult, however, as little as 30 days of deliberately redirecting your thoughts to ones that are more supportive of your goals will create strong new habits of thought.

Providing smokers with knowledge about the personal impact of unhealthy thought processes and skills they can use to modify undesirable patterns will increase their chances of permanently becoming non-smokers.

Smoking is the one risk factor that is 100% preventable. No one has to smoke cigarettes. Many factors contribute to the decision to smoke, which hinder individual efforts to overcome the habit.

We know that smokers are more anxious than non-smokers are and most believe smoking has a calming effect[20]. Most smokers believe they cannot quit when they are under high stress and that even if they quit, their efforts to remain a non-smoker will be negatively impacted if the level of stress in their lives increases[21].

♥ Jeanine Joy
TRUE Prevention—Optimum Health

Twenty-five years ago, I decided to become a non-smoker during what I thought would be the most stressful period of my life. I was glad I was under so much stress at the time because I used the situational stress, and my success at becoming a non-smoker under those circumstances, to convince myself that no matter what I faced in the future, I could do it without returning to what I termed "The Demon Nicotine." I am delighted to report that developing this belief serves me well and even thought I have had periods of even higher stress, I have not returned to smoking.

When I became a non-smoker, I was in college and happened to be taking a class where they had us take a test that used a point system to establish our current level of stress. I was far above the beginning score for the highest stress category. At the time, I answered yes to the following questions:

- Have you gone through a divorce in the past 12 months?
- Have you bought a house during the past 12 months?
- Have you changed jobs during the past 12 months?
- Has your boss changed during the past 12 months?
- Have you had a change in financial circumstances during the past 12 months?
- Have you changed schools in the past 12 months?

There were other stressful events happening simultaneously that were not captured by the survey. I became a non-smoker the week before finals. At the time, I was working full-time managing 24 employees—all of whom were born before me. I was also designing and implementing changes to policies at work due to sweeping industry changes mandated by The Equity and Fiscal Responsibility Act of 1982 (TEFRA)s and the Deficit Reduction Act of 1984 (DEFRA) in a company without a compliance department, an attorney who did not have a life or annuity insurance background, amid an industry full of misinterpretations in the published literature. The stressful changes all occurred within the past six months (not the 12 months the scale measured). My former husbands' sister was my secretary and the new boss

> *Building resilient thought processes leads to pro-health and pro-social outcomes. Thought processes and personality traits are not fixed—they rarely change only because the skills to change them have not been widely understood. Focusing on the risks of smoking may increase anxiety and depression, thus increasing the difficulty of quitting.*

was a man I had left my prior employer to get away from due to his unethical behaviors[22].

For about twenty years, I said that if I ever figured out how I went from a 2-pack a day Marlboro girl to being a non-smoker—meaning if I could explain why it worked so others could replicate it—I would write a book. I am writing that book. This book is not the appropriate place to go into all the details, but the processes described in the last chapters will be very beneficial to anyone wishing to "Beat the Demon Nicotine" for good.

I include my story here because the concept of waiting to quit until the level of stress is lower is a common theme. Quitting when you are under a high level of stress is actually a more powerful statement that will serve anyone who chooses this path well, both in terms of increased ability to maintain the new, non-smoking status and in feeling more empowered and optimistic about their future. To put a more modern spin on the work-stress related to TEFRA and DEFRA, compare it to implementation of the Affordable Care Act.

One of the reasons stressful incidents can lead to relapse for an individual who has quit smoking is that nicotine causes the brain to release beta-endorphin and norepinephrine, which results in temporary improvements in mood. This relationship trains a smoker to rely on cigarettes to improve his mood when he is uncomfortably stressed. Providing stress reducing/happiness increasing skills before she quits increases resistance to relapse due to stressful events. People will choose the path most in alignment with their goals. Using skills to manage stress, instead of cigarettes, will be in greater alignment with their goals.

Smoking can also be a contemplative time. Helping smokers understand that giving themselves that time, without the cigarette, can also be beneficial to long-term success. The higher the stress level, the greater benefit the smoker will feel from taking the time out. When I became a non-smoker, I deliberately continued taking smoke breaks with my friends—to enjoy their company. I had mentally prepared and visualized myself doing this without smoking before I became a nonsmoker. This allowed me to continue the social aspects of smoking that I enjoyed, without the undesired habit.

To summarize, stress has a significant role:
- In the beginning of the habit via peer pressure
- In frequently delaying efforts to quit
- In relapse after having quit
- In increasing the reward a smoker experiences from smoking

Smokeless Tobacco and e-cigarettes

Before we go much further, I wanted to mention that smokeless tobacco is known to cause cancer in humans[23]. Also, e-cigarettes have been introduced without research about their safety. They contain substances known to be harmful to humans including carcinogens.[24] I have met individuals who believe they are beating the system by switching to smokeless tobacco instead of quitting in the mistaken belief that smokeless tobacco will not harm their health.

Chapter 4: Physical Activity

*A stationary bike is a device that
epitomizes the phrase "hurry up and wait."*
Jarod Kintz

Inactivity, or low levels of physical activity, is a risk factor for developing heart disease. There are so many intertwined factors affecting physical activity that it can become convoluted. However, the thread of poor stress management skills is woven throughout.

Physical activity is an area where false premises are commonly believed. This often hinders individuals' efforts to improve or sustain their health at desired levels. For example, the overall outcome of exercise from positive motivation may be significantly better than the same exercise motivated by negative emotion. Let me say that again, in a different way.

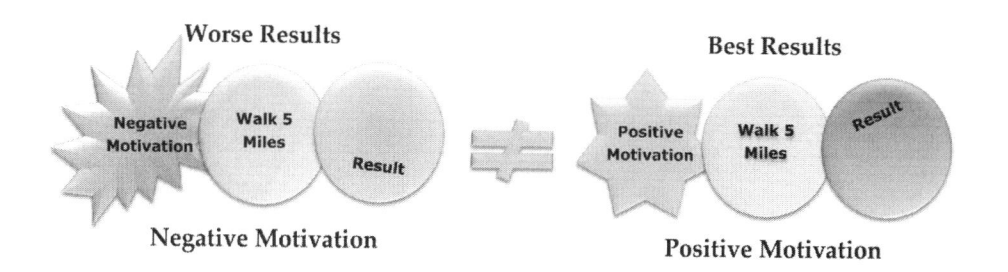

Worse Results — Negative Motivation + Walk 5 Miles = Result
Best Results — Positive Motivation + Walk 5 Miles = Result

Negative Motivation ≠ **Positive Motivation**

If you guilt yourself into running every morning, the health benefits you receive are less than the health benefits you could receive from the same amount of time and action if you used positive methods to motivate yourself. Additionally, using positive motivation lessens the effort required. That may sound confounding. I will explain.

If you're taking a 5-mile walk with the mindset that you don't really want to do it, but because you want to maintain your health, you do it—or you do it to offset the piece of cheesecake you ate the night before, it can feel like you're pushing forward while strapped to heavy weights.

If, on the other hand, you listen to music that makes you want to move—music that makes moving joyful—and look forward to being able to listen to the music without interruption while you walk 5 miles, it can feel as if you're being carried along, easily accomplishing the 5-mile goal.

Because mindset affects our perception, a positively focused mindset lessens the resistance we feel to the activity. Perceptually, it requires less effort. It feels like it requires less effort energetically. For the purposes of this book, I will leave it at the perceptual level. Our perception is what leads to our actual experience.

Exercising because you enjoy moving your body is far healthier than the same exercise done because you fear the consequences of not exercising.

The New Scientific Understanding of Body Weight Management

- Health Status
- Mood Mindset
- Exercise
- Calories
- Stress

Weight (BMI) Health

Mindset Matters

The negative motivation mindset increases stress. Stress causes changes in body chemistry that increase appetite and reduce numerous pro-health behaviors—including exercise.

Wellness programs that use fear (i.e. negative health consequences of low physical activity, smoking, poor diet and obesity) have affects that counter their goals[25]. Negative motivation techniques increase stress and can reduce motivation for pro-health behaviors. For most, the idea that walking five miles does not bestow the same benefits as walking five miles with the variable being the motivation leading to the physical activity is a very new concept. In fact, most people will reject the line of thought as fanciful or impossible.

In Chapter 14, I demonstrate why mindset matters. It has to do with chemical changes that happen in our bodies based on our mindset. For now, I will not ask you to take my word for it. I will ask you to consider the possible consequences by asking yourself "What if this is true?" Please do not close your mind to potentially beneficial information just because it contradicts what you currently believe. That would be the Galileo Effect.

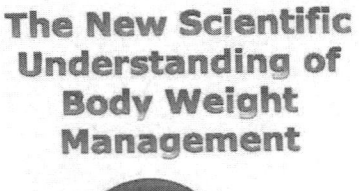

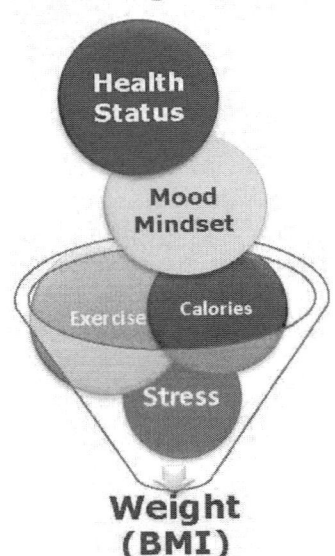

Before a deeper explanation is provided, several common false premises that undermine efforts to increase physical activity will be discussed. The first myth is a common truism about body weight management. Anyone who has struggled with weight issues—either underweight or overweight—will confirm that it seems more complicated than calories in and calories burned. They are right. The old beliefs about weight assumed our bodies were very simplistic machines—almost box-like to the extent it expected that whatever was put in either remained or was burned up to fuel the body.

We all know that our cars, which are far less complex than our bodies, do not operate in this exact way. Some of our cars have higher gas mileage ratings than others. Even the same make, model, and year of vehicle, running on the same fuel, will experience variances in the miles per gallon (MPG) it receives based on factors such as whether the tires are the same or, if they are the same, whether the air pressure in the tires is the same.

Our bodies are far more complex systems than a car. It amazes me that such a simplistic model ever became poplar dogma regarding maintenance of desired weight. Science has now demonstrated that current health status, mood, calories, exercise, and stress level <u>all</u> contribute to body weight management.

Are there additional factors that we do not yet understand? I would feel foolish believing we have all the answers. What I believe we have is more answers than we once did—factors that will help the public understand and accept healthier and more accurate beliefs about weight management.

JUDGMENT AND STRESS

The widely held, but inaccurate, beliefs that individuals whose BMI exceeds normal are lazy or less intelligent or any number of other derogatory beliefs is harmful to both those with excess BMI and to those with normal weight who operate with those beliefs.

> *It was after I first began to uplift my thoughts a bit that my cravings for junk food started to dissipate. I did not connect the two at that time. First, I simply noticed that I did not need to sleep so much. It took a while before I realized that in addition to my improved energy level, there was a direct correlation between chewing on mental garbage and putting garbage in my mouth.*
>
> *Holly Mosier*

You might ask how a belief about something others do can negatively affect the individual with the belief. It has to do with the body chemistry of the person holding an unfavorable viewpoint. When we think of someone and judge him as lacking in some way, we do not feel as good as when we look at someone and judge him as wonderful.

Stay with me—this is not readily apparent to many people. They think the negative emotion they feel when they look at someone else and judge the person as lacking in some way reflects something wrong with the person they are judging. It doesn't.

Think about someone you loved without reservation at some point in your life—perhaps a childhood friend, a new baby, or the first person you fell in love with who loved you back. When you were in that state of mind about that person, you felt great. Right? When you're loving someone in that way the world seems more beautiful—all of life just seems better. Pause for a moment and remember how that felt.

Now, while you are remembering as much of that feeling as possible, ask yourself this, "How much stress did I feel in those moments when I was loving so fully?" The feeling you are looking for is during a moment, day, week, hour—whatever you can find in your memories—when you were purely loving.

The baby was not crying or fussy if you are using a new baby for the memory. Perhaps the baby just gave you her first smile. The memory is not during a time when you were anxious about whether someone loved you nor is it during a disagreement. It is a moment of harmonious love.

Poke around at the memory in your own mind and you'll see your stress level was insignificant during that time of flowing unrestricted love to another person. It felt great. Your body felt strong and energized. You may have wanted it to remain that way forever.

Now compare it to a time when you were judging someone as lacking in some way due to the results of their body weight management. How much stress did you feel in your body as you thought about someone else in that way—even if it was a stranger?

Sometimes judging feels better and sometimes worse, depending on the emotional state you are in when you begin judging. For example, someone who has been thinking unhappily about their own weight management results may feel better when they observe another whose results they judge as even worse than their own. This is even more apparent in some scenarios.

Imagine for a moment that you are going to a school reunion. Perhaps you consider not going because you are more conscious of the weight you have gained since graduation under these circumstances. Your thoughts stray to a rival from that era of your life that may be at the reunion, which adds to your stress.

Fast forward—imagine yourself at the reunion. You spot your rival and notice a weight gain of more pounds than you have gained. In that moment, most people will feel a sense of relief. The concern about being there with extra weight diminishes. You end up having a better time than you would have if your rival looked like a super star.

In this situation, another's weight gain made you feel better. However, I would do you a disservice if I did not point out that this happened from a disempowered perspective. *Using others as the measuring stick to judge our own value leaves us powerless to do anything about the situation.*

Now imagine that you and a friend are enjoying a pleasant conversation while sipping a beverage at a sidewalk café. You are feeling relaxed and are enjoying the beautiful weather. Then you notice someone walking past that is exposing more skin than you prefer to see on someone with that particular body type—destroying your relaxed mood.

You may feel disgust. You may feel jealous (if it is a person who is exhibiting the type of shape you desire). You may feel frustrated. The way you emotionally respond to the stimulus can vary. Focus on the level of stress you would feel before and after the stranger distracts you from the pleasant conversation.

Regardless of whether your emotion is disgust, jealousy, frustration, or some other negative viewpoint, your level of stress increased because of the judgment. In the case of disgust, you are judging the other person as lacking. In jealousy and frustration, you are judging yourself as lacking in comparison.

In your mind, go back to the sidewalk café and imagine that the person you notice is not a stranger. In this scenario, imagine someone you love dearly and wish the best for. If the person you imagined was overweight, imagine that despite being overweight, their current size is a significant improvement from their size the last time you saw them. You are consciously aware that they are moving in the direction of their goals and you feel happy about their progress.

Now notice your stress level during this scenario. It is lower—at least until you begin worrying whether he will be able to continue losing or until you think about the potential negative health impact of the weight he is carrying.

Try another scenario, the person whose magnificent shape led you to feel jealous in the first situation is someone you love who has been going through a divorce—someone who had gained weight during the stressful end of the marriage. As you observe his confident stride, you feel a sense of relief because it is obvious that your friend has achieved a better state of mind about the end of his marriage. Your initial reaction is not jealousy because you are focused on rejoicing about the progress he has made. Your emotions may eventually become jealous as you wish you had made similar changes but that comes later, if at all.

Notice your stress level in this situation. If you have been worried about this friend, you may feel lighter upon seeing him obviously feeling better.

Considering the above scenarios, can you see that it was your thoughts about the situations that generated the emotions you felt? It is your thoughts and perception about situations that determine how much stress you actually experience. We are able to achieve far more control over our habitual thoughts than most understand.

Until now, we were not taught to adjust our thoughts. We were told to take action. Action is important, but unhealthy thinking diminishes the results of the action. Reducing stress increases both the likelihood that an individual will exercise and the benefits they receive from the exercise.

MAKE PLAY OK™ CAMPAIGNS

As I considered the symptom of low physical activity, I was struck by the lessons children are taught that contribute to an unhealthy lack of physical activity as adults. Adult physical activity is negatively impacted by some prevalent beliefs including:

- Play is for kids
- Adults should know everything so they should not fail at anything
- Adults should not look silly
- Demonstrate maturity by sitting still and not fidgeting

Think about most adult physical activity and you will see a predominant belief that exercising involves going to a gym, jogging, or taking long walks whether we want to or not. Physical activity for most adults is not about having fun. Some people enjoy going to a gym. More enjoy the results of going to a gym far more than what they do at the gym.

There are adults who enjoy fun physical activities including kayaking, hiking, baseball, basketball, football, and even running, but most adult physical activity is done with the motivation to fulfill an obligation to maintain one's health, not to have fun. This mindset is detrimental to our health.

Think about what motivates you. If you exercise regularly, how do you explain your reason when asked? If you don't exercise regularly, do you tell yourself you should? Do you mentally beat yourself up for not exercising? Why do you tell yourself you should exercise more? If you are repeatedly telling yourself something like, "You don't exercise enough," or, "You're going to gain weight because you don't exercise enough," or, "If you don't start exercising you're going to die young," you are affirming the undesired. Affirming what you do not want leads to long term self-fulfilling prophesies.

Could you find time to go outside and play? Would you feel comfortable learning a new game? If not, why?

The mechanics of negative self-talk are complex. First, self-criticism increases your level of stress. That causes biochemical changes in your body—including depressing your immune system, reducing your energy, and other stress responses. None of this is healthy for your body. Then, the mind, which is very malleable and obedient to repeated affirmations, forms beliefs that lead to the exact outcomes you are telling yourself you will experience by giving yourself the negative affirmations.

If you are in the habit of negative self-criticism, do everything you can to stop it. Refuting it is a good tool. You can begin by shifting a little bit. For example, "I am learning to reduce my stress level. When my level of stress is lower, I will naturally feel like exercising more. My body enjoys moving and soon I will move it more." This refuting statement may be more than you can believe right now. If that is so, find something you do believe that feels better than the negative self-talk. Take baby steps.

As you learn stress-decreasing skills and your energy level rises, kick it up a little: "I feel more energetic than I used to. I am enjoying adding exercise to my day. My body really enjoys moving. Now I enjoy it, too." Find affirmations that you can believe and that support what you want. If you can't believe anything close to what you want yet, just move in that direction a step at a time. With an unhealthy mindset about ourselves, or aspects of physical activity, we can harm our health by increasing stress:

1. Self-induced stress caused by making exercise about preventing illness.
2. Self-induced stress from negative self-criticism related to not exercising or not doing it well enough or often enough.
3. Stress from peer and parental pressure to act grown-up and forgo fun childish physical activities.

Research has shown the motivation behind physical activity affects the results. The whole mindset that adults do not play (or should not play) does society a great disservice. Playing is fun, it decreases tension (stress), it builds relationships, and it helps us move our bodies from a positive motivational force.

It is acceptable for an adult to use a jump rope at the gym and jump until they are dripping sweat. But, go to a public place and play jump rope and sing:

Teddy Bear, Teddy Bear, turn around
Teddy Bear, Teddy Bear, touch the ground,
Teddy Bear, Teddy Bear, show your shoe,
Teddy Bear, Teddy Bear, that will do!

How silly would you feel jumping rope with other adults and singing this or dozens of other ditties associated with jumping rope? Could you stand to appear that silly in front of other adults? If you were able to get past the silliness of it, would this not be far more fun than jumping rope for the purpose of exercise? Can you imagine walking next door and asking another grown-up to come out and play jump rope with you?

Let me ask you this: Why isn't this okay? Why should we have to put play behind us when we reach adulthood and only exercise in adult approved ways? It is because we worry about what others will think about us—we worry they will perceive us as less adult, or less grown up, than we *should* be.

If we are fulfilling our adult responsibilities, such as working, paying our bills, and being honorable in our relationships, etc., should it matter what someone else thinks? Why would we choose to limit ourselves by forcing ourselves to do physical activity we don't find enjoyable when we could play instead?

Jump rope is not the only option. What about tag? Hide N Go Seek? Volleyball? Lawn games like Lemonade—does anyone else remember this one? In the version played in my neighborhood, we divided the neighborhood kids into two groups or teams. One group lined up along the driveway of the house on the left, the other group would come up with a charade to perform. They would cross the lawn to a point closer to the driveway and act out a hastily thought up play or charade, with great silliness and laughter on all sides. The other team attempted to guess the word being acting out, and when someone guessed the phrase correctly, the acting team immediately turned and attempted to reach the "safety" of the other driveway while the guessing team chased them. Anyone who was tagged had to change teams.

We played until our parents made us come in, until the mosquitoes got too bad, or, on the best nights, until it was too dark to see. The game was fun and involved exercise (sprinting across the lawn) every few minutes. It never seemed like exercise. We played for hours in the summertime. If too many parents called their children home for us to form large enough teams, we would change to playing Hide N Go Seek.

Charades games are popular with adults, but do not involve running. Our society has bundled "being an adult" with restrictions on play. I do not believe it is because adults would not enjoy playing, but that adults do not believe it is publically Okay to play. Campaigns to change this mindset could go a long way to encouraging healthier behavior and stronger communities.

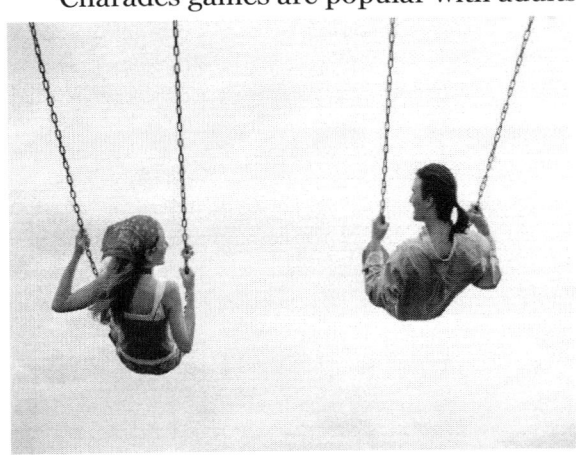

Making Play OK™ is something corporate wellness programs could easily promote. What childhood activities would you still enjoy? I love swinging on a swing set. There are appropriate times to be serious and "grown-up," but we miss many opportunities when playing would be Okay.

The idea that adults should know how to do things keeps many adults who did not have an opportunity to experience things as a child from trying them as adults. Adults who did not learn to skate or swim as children tend not to learn as adults—even when they have the resources to do so—because they are afraid of looking silly.

If we place greater emphasis on the value of learning, even learning new ways to play, instead of on always wanting to appear competent in what we are doing, it would be another beneficial step forward in making play Okay. Yes, we want to be competent in our chosen careers, but insisting we always look that way holds us back from learning new things. There is a learning curve to any new activity, at any age, and it is perfectly Okay to not be as good as someone with experience in the beginning, and remembering this would serve society well in many areas.

Let's redefine what it means to be a grown up. Let's make grown-ups into blended beings who are free to express both a serious nature and a playful nature.

You're it!

Chapter 5: Weight Management

You must begin to think of yourself as becoming the person you want to be.

David Viscott

Stress plays a significant role in body weight management. Chronic stress causes chemical changes in the body that make it hold onto weight. In some people, stress reduces appetite resulting in unhealthy low body weights and poor nutrition. In others, food is the preferred anxiety medication. Positivity and optimism have a positive effect on the choice of foods—increasing consumption of high-fiber and nutritional foods. Lower mood (higher stress) is associated with consumption of higher fat foods[26].

Attempts to modify food related behaviors that do not include modification of habitual stress levels fail in the long-term. Most weight change plans are unsuccessful over the long term. Those that include behavior modification aimed toward reducing stress are the most successful[27]. This makes a great deal of sense when a broader view of weight management is applied.

> *Reducing stress first makes weight change goals easier to attain.*

1. People naturally choose healthier foods when their stress level is low (positively focused).
2. The body's response to food results in healthier outcomes when the stress level is low. When the stress level is high, the body chemistry changes which increases weight retention.
3. Food is frequently used as comfort food during high stress.
4. When stressed, our bodies do not absorb as much nutrition as when we're not stressed, which can lead to constant hunger.

Chapter 5: Weight Management

The willpower needed to stick to a weight management program is significantly higher when the individual is stressed than when in a positive state of mind.

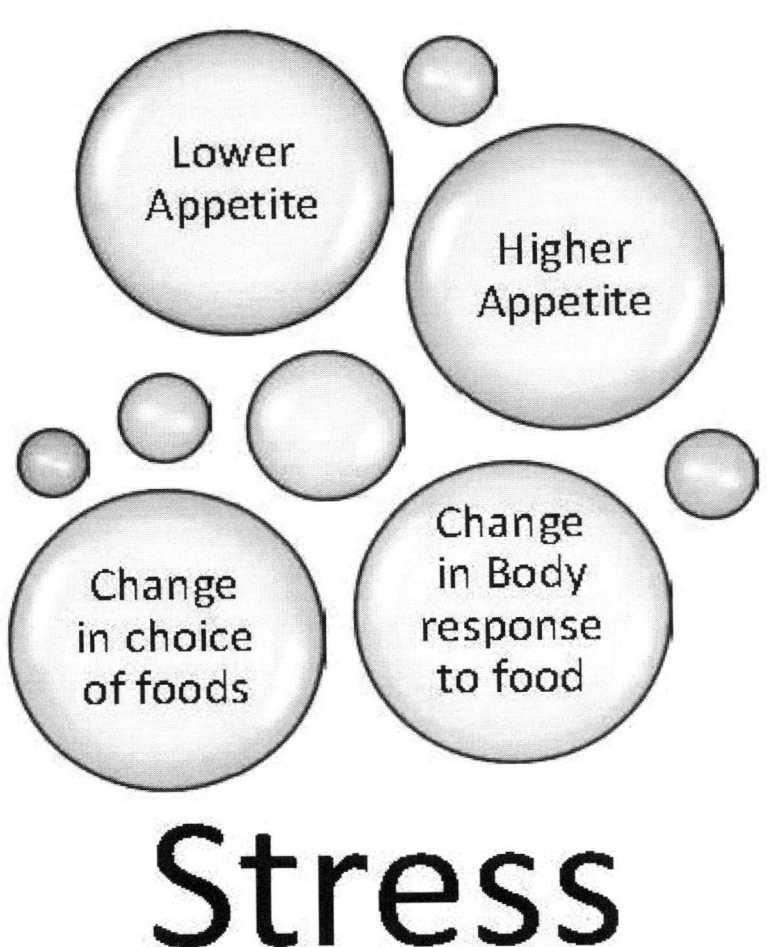

- Lower Appetite
- Higher Appetite
- Change in choice of foods
- Change in Body response to food

Stress

Adverse Weight Judgments

Consider the effect of adverse weight judgments on the level of stress. Regardless of whether we judge others or ourselves, when we find fault or flaws, our stress level increases. This creates unhealthy changes in our body chemistry. I'm going to spend some time providing examples of this because the way the scenario's I'll describe are typically perceived is different from what we need to know to make healthier decisions for ourselves.

If you have ever been overweight, you know you were probably your own worst critic. Others adding their disapproval did not increase your motivation. In fact, research indicates stigmatization reduces individual ability to make desired changes in weight[28]. Supportive attitudes are better for everyone involved.

When society understands the impact of stress on weight management, the response to someone who is gaining weight may become less about the weight and more about what is going on in other areas of their life. If that is done from a supportive perspective, just that change could make the world a nicer place and a healthier place.

For example, I have noticed with my students that there is a strong correlation between excess body weight and a history of abuse. In a study from Stony Brook University in New York, they found that 61% of severely obese individuals reported a history of childhood abuse, 30.5% reported interpersonal abuse as adults, and 15% reported clinically significant depressive symptoms[29]. Disclosure of abuse by my students has usually occurred after they have taken steps to heal the emotional pain and the weight they have struggled to lose for years seems to melt away.

I have also noticed a correlation between heartache and excess weight. Although I am unaware of any research that supports this observation, it is logical. When someone without well-developed stress management skills experiences heartache, gaining weight can be a defensive mechanism. This would be especially true for someone with a tendency to be hard on herself. The last thing this individual needs is criticism from others.

When someone is obviously carrying excess weight, the individual is probably hurting in some way. Compassion is a healthy response. If you see an opportunity to be of benefit, whether with a kind or encouraging word—or more, if the individual seems open to receiving advice—act on it. I do not view the individual as helpless. Be kind, but never make it about the weight—tips on healthy eating are not what the individual needs. Compliment a pretty smile, kindness, intelligence, or their potential in some area.

Weight issues are often a silent plea for help from someone who simply wants to heal but does not know how. There is no shame in not knowing how. Our society has a shroud over emotional pain, as if experiencing it is somehow shameful, to be addressed only behind closed doors on a therapists couch.

A solution can be so much simpler than that for most people. Stress management skills are all many people need to increase their resilience and enjoyment of life. Another false premise prevalent in our society is that holding up under enormous pressure (stress) without breaking—proving our strength--is somehow valiant, a desired state of being. This Stoic attitude kills a lot of people. Unmanaged stress is the root cause of illness and many social ills.

Stress and emotions that do not feel good are not something to be tolerated. In chapter 11, I introduce research that indicates the right response to stress. "Right" is defined as the response that is supportive of our wellbeing.

Although severely underweight individuals receive less public distain, the root can be the same. Often, a conversation quickly reveals the individual is highly stressed—often due to negative self-talk in the privacy of his or her own mind. Chronic stress is insidious to weight management—sometimes resulting in obesity and other times anorexia, bulimia, or an underweight body. One symptom of unmanaged high stress is a weight management issue. It manifests differently with each individual. Some people use food to soothe their anxiety while others feel too nauseated by stress to eat a balanced diet.

It is my hope that this is the last era that will endure such high stress, not because all the world's problems will be resolved and life will be easy, but because current society has not been taught healthy ways to manage stress. Many of our current practices increase the stress burden significantly. The stigma attached to "emotional issues" and many of the symptoms of unmanaged stress such as obesity, smoking, and depression is one way our society exacerbates the problem.

We can do much to be kinder to one another. In making the choice to be kinder we will actually advance our own desires further. Many obese individuals report having experienced verbal abuse and teasing related to their weight. Sadly, they often point to their own families as the source of the worst of it. The family members' good intentions backfire because they do not realize chronic stress is the root cause of the problem and their behavior creates additional stress.

Stress management training includes helping individuals refute negative and hurtful comments from others in the privacy of their own minds. The power the comments have to hurt is up to the way they are perceived. It is possible to understand that the reason someone is being harsh about one's weight is because he cares about us. We can focus on the fact that he cares, instead of the dysfunctional manner in which the message is relayed.

It is not necessary to change the other's actions or to object to the way he expresses his worry. That sort of response usually does not help and often results in deterioration of the relationship. We can change how we receive the message to eliminate the sting. Learning to respond from a lower stress level will facilitate our own desire to manage our weight.

In the area of weight management there is a growing movement that, when considered in light of what we know, is misguided. This pertains to a growing call for the prohibition of junk food. Limiting junk food, especially for children, seems wise. Banning "junk food" does not seem like a wise move. First, there is the strong evidence that food choices are affected more by mood than by education—especially when the stress level is high. The saying, "Food is the most commonly used anxiety drug" should be considered. What are other common ways individuals address anxiety? Alcohol, drugs, smoking, and shopping all come to mind. You might think shopping is innocuous, but consider the personal debt load in this country. Consider what we know and you are learning in this book about the detrimental effect of stress (worry) on our health and relationships and you'll quickly see the correlation between shopping as a habitual response to stress for the negative implications it has on health.

Eating is a better response than some other choices. If we eliminate junk food as an option, would more people turn to shopping, alcohol, or drugs? What about the underground market? History is clear about what happened when alcohol was criminalized. It pushed the consumption of alcohol into speakeasies and created a new criminal element. It also removed alcohol taxes as a revenue source and into a cost to society for the efforts to discover the stills hidden in the woods. Some of my ancestors had a still in Tennessee. When I visited in 1984, they still made home brew because they could avoid the alcohol taxes.

Drugs are another area where, unless prescribed by a physician, there is an underground and criminal economy. The evidence of what happens when something people desire is illegal is clear. The advocates of a prohibition against junk food are missing the big picture.

It is not a lack of knowledge about what is healthy that makes individuals consume junk food. I know what I should eat. I also know that if I allow myself to become stressed out, a bag of BBQ potato chips is in my future (not the whole bag). That is my stressed out food. I know dozens of ways to feel less stressed, but sometimes my old stoicism habits and determination to finish some (usually arbitrary) deadline I've established for myself increase my stress level to a point where I feel I do not have time to eat and the potato chips call my name. Even consciously recognizing that I should take a break and make something healthy, go for a walk, or meditate to get my head in a better place, I chose the chips. If they weren't available, would I turn to fruit or vegetables? Probably not. I would feel worse because someone is controlling my personal decisions and infringing on my personal freedom. That could make my solution a glass of wine. I might also decide to buy the

> *It is as important to be picky about what we allow in our minds, as it is what we consume.*

products in an underground market (which would be created in response to the demand if such foods were criminalized).

The relationship between stress and body weight management is significant. Stress:

- Reduces the likelihood that healthy foods will be selected
- Changes the body chemistry, resulting in the body holding on to unwanted pounds
- Can lead to eating disorders
- Increases consumption of comfort foods with low nutritional value
- Can make people too nauseous to eat
- Can lead to over consumption
- Can increase appetite

Although healthy weight management is affected by our choices, our choices are affected by stress. Long-term efforts to solve unhealthy weight management usually fail. Addressing the underlying stress, will prevent significant numbers of weight management issues and help those who are currently struggling to make improvements.

Chapter 6: Nutrition

The Harvard Law states: Under controlled conditions of light, temperature, humidity, and nutrition, the organism will do as it damn well pleases.
Larry Wall

While education about nutrition is important, our conversation should not stop there. Most people can differentiate between healthy and unhealthy food choices, yet during times of high stress, they will make the unhealthy choice. Facts about healthy food choices are insufficient to benefit most people when they are stressed or overly tired. Food is the most frequently used anxiety drug.

It is not possible to separate emotion from food. Anyone who attempts to do so is fooling himself. When discussing the nutritional value of food, we focus almost exclusively on what we've been taught about which foods are unhealthy, and which ones are healthy. When we choose comfort foods to assuage our stress, self-criticism and/or disappointment in our self, about the food choice can increase our level of stress. Willpower plays a minor role in our food choices, stress plays the most important role; affecting both, our choice of foods and our body's ability to derive the most benefit and fewest adverse effects from the foods we choose. Goals, habits, and intentions play a larger role than willpower.

Setting goals for healthy eating can help individuals be more aware of their choices as they make them. Setting intentions may seem inherent in goal setting, but a deliberate reinforcement of ones intentions makes it more likely we will adhere to self-imposed goals. Without a strong intention, goals function more like a wish list for some individuals. Good eating habits can be developed regardless of past food choices. Being more aware of the choices we make helps us develop healthier habits.

It is easy to go into the grocery store and put familiar items in our cart. Plan to take more time, read labels, learn about the foods you have been choosing. Explore information foods you have not tried. Take your smart phone and look up the nutritional value of fruits and vegetables. I find it helpful to use online tools to research the nutritional information of foods and keep a single page chart of the healthiest choices in my purse. Not all fruits and vegetables are created equal. Also, pay attention to how you feel after you eat various foods. Keeping a food journal one week each season for a year can provide you with significant insights about foods that may be sabotaging your goals.

Stress management training will do far more to increase healthy food choices than repeated education about the right choices. Even though I will still turn to BBQ potato chips when I am highly stressed, the effect of stress management training is that my stress level only reaches the comfort food stage about 4% of what it used to. The number of times an individual does not reach for the comfort food because the circumstances that would have caused the comfort food response in the past simply do not generate the same degree of stress. Well-developed stress management skills allow me to keep my stress below the level where I reach for comfort foods.

Outside circumstances, such as my daughter being in an accident, a lay-off, the ending of a relationship, or someone I care about being seriously ill no longer trigger the potato chip response. It is only when I push myself too far on what I want to accomplish in a set timeframe that I allow myself to become both stressed and fatigued that I reach for comfort foods. Like everyone, I am a work-in-progress. I expect to continue improving.

Speaking of fatigue, we seriously overlook the role fatigue has on stress. A level of stress managed with equanimity when rested might lead to serious difficulties when overtired.

I am not going to list which foods are healthy and how much we should eat of which type. That information is freely available on the internet, taught in schools, and frequently changed. What I want to talk about in the area of nutrition is the connection between how we feel and the food choices we make. I also want to talk about how food is processed differently by our bodies when we are in different emotional states.

The Harvard meta-analysis that demonstrated positivity and optimism reduce the risk of heart disease by 50% also found that we make better (healthier) choices about what we eat when we are in a good mood. Once again, stress management skills matter. If individuals manage their personal stress levels to the low stress, high positivity side of the continuum, they naturally make healthier decisions about what to eat.

When we feel bad, we make much poorer choices about what we eat.

The current paradigm ignores how we feel and tells us to use willpower to make the right decisions regarding nutrition. If we just get happy, we will make the good choices without willpower. The willpower route has several drawbacks. One, it is not easy to sustain. Two, we are fighting against our bodies and ourselves. Our body chemistry is different when we feel good—in a way that makes the same foods more beneficial to us than they are when we are in a poor mood.

> Just imagine, how much easier our lives would be if we were born with a 'user guide or owner's manual' which could tell us what to eat and how to live healthy.
> Erika M. Szabo

Like the overtired child who clings to its mother, when we are in low emotional states, our bodies cling to the food we eat and store it as fat. Erika Szabo's quote wishes for a "user guide" that directs us toward what food choices to make in order to be healthy. The truth is we do have a user guide. The reason we do not know we have one is we were taught to misinterpret its messages. I will provide information the reader can use to learn how to interpret their guidance accurately.

Nutrition is important and eating healthy foods is important, but the less stressed people feel while they eat, the more nutrition is absorbed. Some of us use foods to celebrate. For us, happy times may increase our food intake. One way to address this is to find another form of celebration. Another way is to substitute healthier choices. Establishing fun, new customs will benefit generations to come. Tastes can be associated with holidays and without those flavors, the holiday may feel incomplete.

Unfortunately, most of those associations are not with healthy foods. Marshmallow bunnies, malted milk ball eggs, and coconut cake at Easter, Caramel apples on Halloween, homemade ice cream on the 4th of July, cookies at Christmas, and pie on Thanksgiving are common food/holiday associations. Last year we substituted a large bowl of fresh berries for the pie at Thanksgiving, and I did not feel deprived because fresh berries are better than pie. If the absence of a certain food would be felt too strongly, make less of the unhealthy food with the holiday association and add a healthy and appealing choice to the menu. The generation that has the strongest association will be satisfied, while younger generations will begin associating the healthier food with the holiday. Think about the long-term when you plan family celebrations.

Do you want your grandchildren to eat the same foods you eat when they entertain their grandchildren? What are your food celebration associations? What substitutes could be made that would not leave you feeling as if you missed out? What about frequent eating habits? Do you habitually eat potato chips during your favorite TV show? Could you substitute berries or fruit? Do you reach for a candy bar in the midafternoon? Would a healthy yogurt work instead?

Try to make small changes at a time without self-criticism about what you used to do. If you stress about what you eat, the outcome is worse. It is not necessary to condemn old habits before you decide to adopt new ones. See it as a learning, growing experience rather than fixing a problem. Make changes because you are evolving into more of who you want to be, not because who you have been in the past was bad. Do you see the difference in the mental attitude between the two? Do you feel how that difference lessens the stress you feel?

Research has shown that just like with exercise, how we feel when we eat affects how our body processes the food. Eating while we feel good is far healthier for us than eating the same foods when we feel bad. Stress impacts not only the choices we make about food, but also how our bodies process the food.

Chapter 7: Depression

When we are true to ourselves, all that is toxic and burdensome simply falls away.

Dina Hansen

Depression is in the Powerless Zone on the emotional guidance scale that I introduce in Chapter 11. The stress of feeling powerless is insidious—it robs us of motivation. It makes life seem hopeless. The current rate of depression (globally) is 350 million people of all ages[30]. In the US alone, the health care costs for depression for adults were 22.8 billion in 2009.

No one wants to stay depressed, but in that emotional state, it can be hard to think of a thought that feels even slightly better. In Chapter 17, a process that is ideal for this emotional state is provided. You also learn about a process that is often recommended to people suffering from depression that is counterproductive when in this emotional state.

Some people will insist that depression is the result of a chemical imbalance in the brain. I will not, and could not dispute that depressed individuals may have a chemical imbalance in their brains. I will not accept the imbalance as the root cause of most depression. The following quote demonstrates beautifully how depression sneaks up on the individual who leaves chronic stress unmanaged:

"All depression has its roots in self-pity, and all self-pity is rooted in people taking themselves too seriously."

At the time Switters had disputed her assertion. Even at seventeen, he was aware that depression could have chemical causes.

"The key word here is roots," Maestra had countered. "The roots of depression. For most people, self-awareness and self-pity blossom simultaneously in early adolescence. It's about that time that we start viewing the world as something other than a whoop-de-doo playground, we start to experience personally how threatening it can be, how cruel and unjust. At the very moment when we become, for the first time, both introspective and socially conscientious, we receive the bad news that the world, by and large, doesn't give a rat's ass. Even an old tomato like me can recall how painful, scary, and disillusioning that realization was. So, there's a tendency, then, to slip into rage and self-pity, which if indulged, can fester into bouts of depression."

"Yeah but Maestra - "

"Don't interrupt. Now, unless someone stronger and wiser - a friend, a parent, a novelist, filmmaker, teacher, or musician - can josh us out of it, can elevate us and show us how petty and pompous and monumentally useless it is to take ourselves so seriously, then depression can become a habit, which, in turn, can produce a neurological imprint. Are you with me? *Gradually, our brain chemistry becomes conditioned to react to negative stimuli in a particular, predictable way. One thing'll go wrong and it'll automatically switch on its blender and mix us that black cocktail, the ol' doomsday daiquiri, and before we know it, we're soused to the gills from the inside out. Once depression has become electrochemically integrated, it can be extremely difficult to philosophically or psychologically override it; by then it's playing by physical rules, a whole different ball game.* [Emphasis added] That's why Switters my dearest, every time you've shown signs of feeling sorry for yourself, I've played my blues records really loud or read to you from The Horse's Mouth. And that's why when you've exhibited the slightest tendency toward self-importance, I've reminded you that you and me - you and I: excuse me - may be every bit as important as the President or the pope or the biggest prime-time icon in Hollywood, but none of us is much more than a pimple on the ass-end of creation, so let's not get carried away with ourselves. Preventive medicine, boy. It's preventive medicine."

Tom Robbins, Fierce Invalids Home from Hot Climates

I do not agree completely with the self-pity and taking oneself too seriously aspects of this quote, but the way the chemical changes take root is more eloquently written than I am currently able to manage. I do agree, completely, that everyone is important. Depression is more difficult when the physical body has been trained to respond to adverse circumstances in a certain way, but it can be overcome. It is amazing how much progress can be made when one-step is taken at a time.

I've already referenced how our mood affects our body chemistry—it can make exercise and food either more or less beneficial. It affects our immune system.[31] In the field of epigenetics, the idea that we are born with certain genealogical tendencies that play out in life has been overthrown. They have seen how a change to a more positive environment has a positive impact on the health and intelligence of mice, not just the one mouse—but up to eight generations of future mice. They have seen that genetic markers turn off and on depending on environment—with emotional state being one of the environmental influencers.

I reject the concept of a chemical imbalance causing depression in isolation. Prolonged chronic stress and/or a major stressful event must play a part in almost every case of depression. If we begin addressing chronic stress in a healthier way, the epidemic levels of depression will be greatly reduced. If all the cases with unmanaged chronic stress as the root cause are eliminated, we'll see more clearly any that have other origins, which will speed solutions for them. Good stress management has the ability to address both prolonged chronic stress and a major stressful event. As you will see in subsequent chapters, the way we perceive an event determines how stressful the event is to our minds and bodies. We have far greater control over how we perceive events than most realize.

Stress control that attempts to control situations does not work. Life happens. We become attached to people and things. We suffer losses and disappointments. Depression is at epidemic levels. The estimates vary between 6.8% to 10% of the population experiencing symptoms of depression in any given year and over half of the population experiencing it during their lifetime. New research indicates depression is a risk factor for teen pregnancy.

Depression has its direct costs to an employer and health care system as an illness. It also carries many other costs. Cognitive abilities diminish as emotional state decreases. The same employee is not capable of the same level of thinking when depressed as she is when not depressed. The same employee is not capable of the same level of thinking when stressed as he is when he is not stressed. What is being lost because an employee is too stressed to see the perfect solution to your company's biggest issues? What is not being invented because the person who could imagine the solution is too stressed to think at the required level?

If we are looking at 100 people with depression and two of them are not caused by chronic stress—but we don't know that because the stress is not managed—we're really studying 98 people who do not have what it is we're attempting to cure and two that are. We will not make much progress until the 98 who can be cured with stress management skills are moved out of the sample.[32]

With depression, even chronic depression, the majority of people who are suffering would benefit greatly from stress management training. Depression affects the depressed individual, their family, and their employer. Productivity losses for depression are estimated at 33%. [33]

Anxiety is closely linked to depression, but because it does not meet the criteria of full blown depression, clinicians may view patients with anxiety as overly worried and miss seeing it as an early treatable symptom of CVD[34].

The suffering is optional. Let's stop taking that option.

Chapter 8: Bits and Pieces

The fact that an opinion has been widely held is no evidence whatever that it is not utterly absurd.
Bertrand Russell

Chronic stress exacerbates the symptoms of cardiovascular disease significantly. Until chronic stress is managed, it is difficult (if not impossible) to eliminate unmanaged stress as the cause of the six symptoms that are commonly considered risk factors for CVD.

While the first seven chapters focused on Cardiovascular (heart) Disease and symptoms thereof, other illnesses and undesired behaviors, which are negatively affected by stress, are worth mentioning. This section will briefly describe a number of them.

> In every area, the findings are essentially the same: reduced stress, which is increased positivity and optimism, is healthier than increased stress and pessimism.

I am not going into great detail in any area because the findings become somewhat boring and redundant after a while. There are so many areas of life including health, relationships, behavior, and success where unmanaged stress has a significant detrimental effect. However, I think it is important to highlight the breadth of the areas where lives are diminished as the result of chronic stress. It provides insight into why I am so passionate about sharing the solutions (stress management techniques that consistently provide relief).

ADDICTIONS

Not all addictions are rooted in abuse or trauma, but I do believe they can all be traced to painful experience. A hurt is at the centre of all addictive behaviours. It is present in the gambler, the Internet addict, the compulsive shopper and the workaholic. The wound may not be as deep and the ache not as excruciating, and it may even be entirely hidden—but it's there. As we'll see, the effects of early stress or adverse experiences directly shape both the psychology and the neurobiology of addiction in the brain.
Gabor Maté

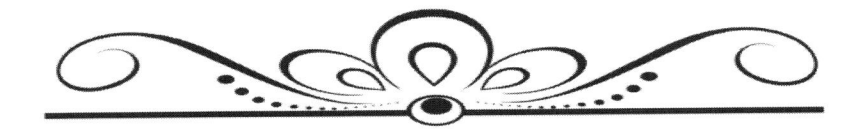

Many factors come into play in addictions. I am not going to delve deeply into the chemical aspects of addictions. To me, they are one of the trees that keep us from seeing the forest. It is good to know they are there, and if we are attempting to develop a drug to counteract the addiction, it is beneficial to understand the details. For our purposes, it is not. Although beneficial drugs could be used in combination with our program, they are not essential to the processes that prevent addiction and relapse.

The onset of addiction stems from stress. I will explain this in several scenarios. Let's begin with a fairly broad picture. In this picture, an individual does not feel good and wants to feel better. For purposes of this illustration, the cause of the unhappiness is irrelevant. The individual then uses alcohol, or a drug, and feels better. We all want to feel better. It does not matter if we are desperately unhappy or pretty happy, the desire to feel even better is always there. It is human nature and it serves great purposes when we follow our guidance.

Because the alcohol or drugs made the person feel better, the next time they want to feel better they may consider it a viable option. Repeat this often enough and a habitual way of addressing stress with an addiction develops. For an individual who has not learned good stress management skills, this may be the best option to feeling better (from that perspective). Even as he begins experiencing a lot of pain from the consequences of his addiction, such as loss of a job, divorce, loss of custody of his children, loss of material possessions, and more—he will not give it up for long because it is the only way he knows to feel emotionally better (or numb the pain).

Addiction is a complex subject. The body's response to the introduction of chemicals (whether from foreign substances such as drugs or alcohol, or more natural mood-enhancing cocktails of serotonin, endorphins, dopamine, phenylethamine, ghrelin, or oxytocin) creates an addictive loop. The individual feels less positive emotion than desired, participates in the addictive behavior, feels the better feelings (or mutes the bad ones).

Typical attempts to attack the addiction focus on ending the chemical addiction. The root cause of the addiction is not typically eliminated. So, if the individual overcomes the addiction and frees herself from it, unless healthy stress management skills have been developed, the risk of relapse is tremendous. The desire to feel better will not go away. Drugs can mute it, but it is still present. Teaching every child how to manage stress and feel good naturally, without unhealthy addictive behaviors, is an achievable and affordable option now.

The same stress management skills would greatly reduce the relapse rate for addicts who successfully complete rehabilitation for the chemical aspect of their addiction.

The initial stress can come from a multitude of situations and circumstances. It could be from peer pressure. Let's address peer pressure for a moment. Peer pressure is pressure from peers that creates stress to go along with what the peer wants. It works when the stress from agreeing is less than the stress of resisting. If a child has been given stress management skills, the path of least resistance to reducing the stress will not be to disobey his parents and go along with peers who want him to try a drug he really does not want to try. It will be to use the stress management skills to reduce the pressure—a far healthier response than taking a drug. The beginning of the addiction cycle can be avoided altogether—true prevention.

The initial stress can come from a multitude of circumstances—it could be studying for law exams, or moving to a new city or country, it could be the end of a relationship, memories of or ongoing abuse, or some other sort of disappointment. Unhealthy habits of thought in the untrained mind such as rumination[35], self-criticism, and catastrophizing often increase the stress felt in such circumstances. These habits increase the negative emotions and create situations in which the individual really needs relief. Alcohol and drugs are, unfortunately, more well-known solutions to high stress than stress management skills.

Many generations have believed that what we think is true. It may be—it may not be. What is true is that we have the ability to think about any situation from a vast number of alternative perspectives; some of them feel good and some don't. We have the ability to deliberately choose to take a perspective that feels better to us—without changing the actual circumstances. This is not suppression; it is a healthy form of adjusting ones perspective.

In fact, if you think about someone you've known whom often seemed upset, you probably noticed that the perspective that person took toward situations in her life was not the same one you would have taken in like circumstances. We notice this and then we (often) attack the individual's choice of perspective. Unless and until an individual understands she has the ability to deliberately shift her perspectives, this tactic will be unproductive and may damage the relationship. In reality, both perspectives are usually equally valid. The angle from which the situation is being viewed determines how it is perceived.

- Let's use being laid off from a job as an example. Here are some examples (by no means a complete list) of perceptions individuals could use to create meaning from the experience.
- I'm a loser. Nothing I try ever works out well for me. (Catastrophizing)
- It was a dumb job anyway. I hope the company gets what it deserves. (Petulant)
- I was ready for a bigger challenge anyway. This is a good opportunity for me to find a better position. (Hopeful, positive expectation)
- I don't know what I'm going to do. That was all I knew how to do and all the jobs are moving to China. I might as well give up. (Depressed)
- Why did I choose to work there in the first place? I could have done something else. Why didn't I? (Self-blame)
- Why did they keep X and let me go? I have way more experience than she does. They have wronged me by doing this. How could they do this to me after all these years? (Anger)
- Every time I get laid off I get a better job making more money. I wonder what is coming my way? (Excited expectation)
- I'm going to make them pay. They don't have the right to do this to me. (Vengeful)
- Maybe this is my chance to go back to school. I think I would enjoy doing X instead of what I've been doing. (Content)
- If I'd just done better on that last project I'm sure they would have kept me. (Guilt)
- If management ran the company better, the lay-offs would not have been necessary. (Blame)

All of the above are valid ways of perceiving the situation. Before you disagree with the "excited expectation" example as far too optimistic, I will self-disclose that that was my exact response to being laid off in 2006 and 2009. I deliberately cultivated and reinforced this mindset after my first lay-off in 2001 turned out so well. I was able to maintain the positive mindset throughout the economic downturn. The reality that followed those lay-offs exceeded my expectations.

Think back to the 2007 – 2012 timeframe and whether you were living in fear of losing your job. For some, it became a reality. Far more people lived in fear of a lay-off than those who experienced one. Many individuals lived diminished years of their lives simply because they focused themselves into a state of fear. Fear diminishes our cognitive abilities, which probably led to more than one self-fulfilling prophesy as work performance declined because of the fear.

Most of the workforce perceives their job security as dependent on their employer. This makes them susceptible to economic changes that negatively affect the organization or industry. My perspective is a more empowered one. I consider myself—my skills, knowledge, and abilities—my job security. As long as I develop me, I am an asset to my employer and will be able to easily find another position. Individuals who strive to make the most of themselves are employable in down economies.

Stress management skills give an individual the ability to choose perspectives that feel better. It does not matter which perspective the individual has in the beginning—all of them are along a continuum. The individual simply chooses one that feels a little better that he can believe from his current perspective. Once the new perspective is adopted, one that is slightly better than the current belief will begin to feel believable. The process can be repeated indefinitely. The individual whose stance was depressed in my examples could, in time, have a highly positive expectation in similar circumstances.

> *How you feel today does not limit how you can feel tomorrow.*

The starting point does not determine the outcome. Consistent application of the process determines the outcome. It is easy to see that moving from the guilt perspective to the blame might feel better. Each step feels better—which provides intrinsic motivation for individuals who know the process to apply it.

Individual who manage themselves into positive emotional states do not need to self-medicate with alcohol or drugs because they already feel good. Another argument those who have not tried the process make is that it depends on other circumstances. They argue someone able to achieve a positive state of mind because their circumstances are less dire—perhaps they do not need the money or have other means of providing for their needs.

I'll do some more self-disclosure using the 2009 layoff as my example. I pick that one because the economy was worse than it was in 2006. In 2009, I was single with two children in college—a freshman and a sophomore, my obligations included a significant mortgage, a car payment, and all the bills associated with modern life. When I was laid-off, I was also booked on two trips—one to Australia and a Panama cruise. I considered, briefly, whether I should cancel the trips and decided that I would find a way to make it work.

In one way, the naysayers are right about the circumstances being different. Identical circumstances are perceived very differently when one believes she will find a way to overcome obstacles and when she believes the situation is hopeless. The circumstances are the same—but the mental attitude makes them feel very differently. The mental attitude, in turn, affects the outcome.

The reason, from my perspective, that relapses are so insidious is not the chemical dependency, it is the desire to feel better by an individual who has not been taught the skills to manage his emotional stance.

Stress management skills help individuals maintain a state of equanimity. It does not take extreme willpower to resist a relapse when someone is able to consciously adjust her perspective to reduce the stress being experienced. Stress management skills are powerful tools for the prevention of addiction and for reducing the likelihood of relapse.

Type II Diabetes

Stress is the trash of modern life-we all generate it but if you don't dispose of it properly, it will pile up and overtake your life.

Danzae Pace

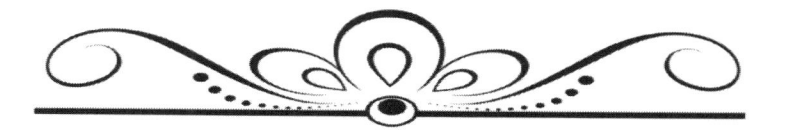

Although Type II Diabetes (I will refer to it hereinafter as simply diabetes) is not one of the six main symptoms of Cardiovascular Disease, it is firmly on the heart disease continuum. There is a strong connection between diabetes and heart disease. The suggestions for preventing CVD throughout this book apply equally to prevention of Diabetes.

What I have written about the "risk factors" of cardiovascular disease in Chapters 1 – 7 applies in much the same way to the development of diabetes. The chapter on Chronic Stress (another significant precursor to diabetes) is in Chapter 16, so that the methods of reducing stress introduced in the intervening chapters can be incorporated in the discussion.

Research into diabetes shows a strong link between unmanaged chronic stress and onset of diabetes.[36] A strong link between diabetes and obesity also exists. Understanding the new way weight management is defined, and especially the interaction between mood and stress, can help millions prevent this disease from disrupting their lives. The Make Play OK™ campaign addresses increased physical activity, which will also help prevent diabetes.

Positivity and optimism have been shown to provide a protective stance against diabetes. Remembering the continuum where unmanaged stress is at one end and happiness (positivity) on the other, we can see this relationship more clearly.

Diabetes is an expensive disease measured in many ways—suffering and loss of vitality, premature mortality, loss of productivity, and direct costs of 176 billion annually.[37]

Everyone, including children, should be taught stress management skills. For the multitude with prediabetes, stress management training has the potential to prevent the majority of them from ever developing the full-fledged disease. This is not only good for those with prediabetes; it would also greatly improve the healthcare economics in this country (and the world) due to the reduction in costs for this expensive disease.[38]

The evidence that unmanaged stress is the root cause of most illness is becoming more evident almost daily. This is definitely the case with diabetes. Providing the information and skills in this book empowers individuals with completely new ways of preventing diabetes.

COGNITION

We now understand that higher-level thinking is more likely to occur in the brain of a student who is emotionally secure than in the brain of a student who is scared, upset, anxious, or stressed.

Mawhinney and Sagan

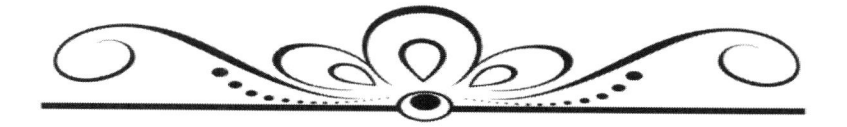

I would be remiss if I did not mention the cognitive benefits of positivity. The same individual is literally smarter when he is positively focused and less intelligent when he is negatively focused. At first, this sounds like rubbish to most individuals. That is only because we have been taught that each person has a certain level of intelligence and most of us still believe that level is immutable. Even though, in many instances, life has shown us the truth of this, we have not connected the dots.

Most of us have either been in a situation, or known someone, who was so distraught that they placed their head in their hands and uttered, "Give me a minute; I can't think."

From both an employer and personal standpoint, increased cognitive ability may be the greatest benefit of positivity. Even in the face of a serious health crisis—the ability to think and find solutions matters. I'll use the example of someone close to me. Two years ago, her cardio doctor told her not to bother fixing her heart—that her lung problems would kill her before her heart would. He was essentially telling her to be hopeless. Instead, he pissed her off—an emotion far better than hopelessness. Since that time, she has had her heart fixed. Through her own efforts and research, she found a study that could fix her specific problem. Now her pulmonary doctor is so impressed with her condition her overall prognosis is greatly improved.

If she had taken that doctor at his word, she would probably be dead by now. If she had felt hopeless, she would never have found a solution because she would not

Keep this in mind when your employees are working on a critical problem. If they are too browbeaten to feel good about finding a solution, the narrowed cognitive abilities may ensure they do not find one.

have even looked. And, at the cognitive level of hopelessness, even if someone else told her of a potential path to feeling better, she would have dismissed it as not beneficial to her. That is how narrowing of cognitive abilities detrimentally affects individuals at the lower end of the emotional scale.

A solution-focused mindset is great for life in general; in crises, it is literally lifesaving. Do you jump on an employee who arrives to work late? Consider that the employee may already be harder on herself than you could ever be. As you fan the flames, you are almost assuring that she will be in a lower emotional state for the rest of the day—with the attendant tendency to make mistakes.

Contrast that with the good you could do with simple understanding, "I know you did everything you could to be here on time today. I know you know how important it is. I'm also sure you've probably learned something today—if there was anything you could have changed—and you'll make adjustments to avoid it in the future." For someone who is already beating up on herself, this would increase her emotional state, making her a more valuable employee that day. Of course, habitual tardiness is another matter—but for the occasional late arrival, it is worth considering this uplifting approach.

Yes, this approach may be counter to what you experienced as an employee. Look deeper at the results and decide for yourself if the old ways makes sense in light of what we now know about the connection between mood and cognitive ability. A choice between a tardy employee who is in a bad mood all day and a tardy employee who is in a good mood is the choice. It is no longer a choice between an employee who arrived on time and one who was tardy. Once the employee is late, the choice you are making is different. A kinder approach does not mean repeated tardiness is OK, or that it will be tolerated indefinitely. Being kind to someone who is tardy does not mean you must allow unlimited tardiness.

Being positively focused is being solution focused.

The lower cognitive abilities are also present when someone is ill or overly tired. I learned this the hard way—going to work when I was ill and making a mistake. When the mistake was discovered, the fact that I had been at work attempting to be a "good employee" by coming to work when I was ill was irrelevant. This was before the risk to other employee's health from presenteeism was viewed as it is today.

When a problem arises, it is possible to look for the silver lining and the opportunities inherent in it. They are always there. The solution-oriented employee is more likely to see them quickly.

Although lowered health care costs and absenteeism are wonderful benefits from stress management skills training, the potential of that one brilliant idea can be of much greater value to an employer than all the savings. The right idea at the right time can generate enough revenue to pay for all the employees' health care, not just their insurance premiums.

On the flip side, one mistake averted can be worth millions. I would love to see someone research some of the great business blunders and the mood/mindset at the time. I'd be willing to bet there is a strong correlation between a low mood and costly blunders.

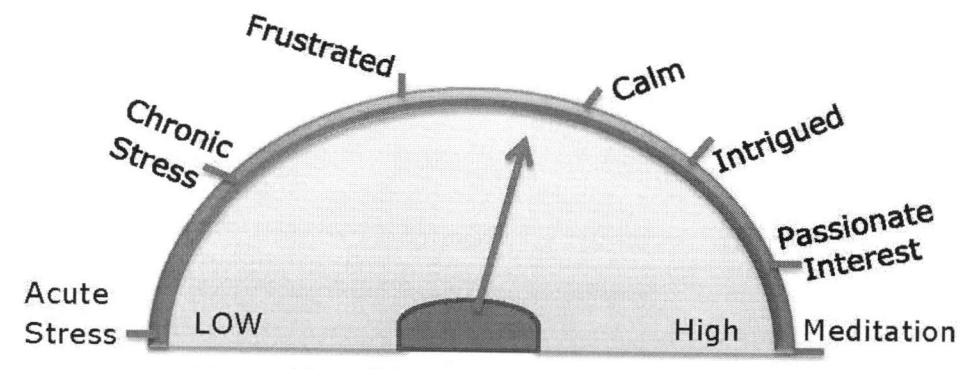

Cognitive Ability: Effect of Stress

There is a commercial where a stressed man in an airport waiting area and seems does not notice another gentleman who attempts to catch his attention—they are wearing the same tie. The stressed man is oblivious to the gentleman attempting to get his attention, so the second gentleman moves to another seat. The screen flashes a message that the value of the deal the stressed man did not get because would have been worth millions.

The next place the second gentleman sits, he is wearing the same socks as another man who does notice him. They begin a friendly conversation, leaving the viewer with the impression that the person who was open to his environment was going to benefit from the interaction.

Although it is a commercial, it reflects real life. The stressed person is often oblivious to opportunities that could resolve the issue that has him stressed. Their brain simply does not connect the dots while they are focused on the problem. Being in a state of mind that is open to opportunity allows us to recognize and harvest those opportunities.

Where are you on the stress meter? Where are your employees?

COLDS AND FLU

I noticed that I would catch a cold when my body was tired of being ignored when it told me it needed a rest.
Unknown

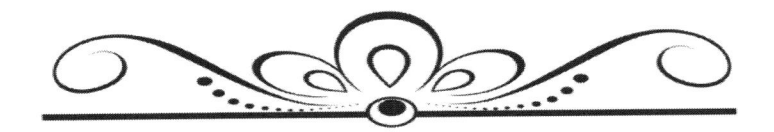

Serious illnesses can seem remote to healthy individuals, like something they will be concerned about someday. Most people have experienced a cold or the flu so it is easier for them to relate to the benefits of positivity when those illnesses are used as an example.

One study in particular demonstrated the benefit of positivity due to its immune function increasing in a very clear way. The study controlled for a number of factors that indicate the relationship between positivity and susceptibility to colds and flu. The researchers measured the degree of positivity the subjects of the research had using standardized tests. During the study, they measured how ill the participants were using two measures. One was to have the participant's journal their symptoms. As expected, the pessimists reported more discomfort and more symptoms of illness.

The researchers also measured the actual output. For example, used tissues were weighed to determine the actual symptoms, temperatures were taken, and other objective measures were taken.

Each participant in the study was deliberately exposed to the virus. The participants were then housed and supervised in separate rooms of a hotel for a week during the study.

As expected, the pessimists reported worse symptoms than the optimists did. The study found that the pessimists were actually sicker than the optimists were. In fact, some of the optimists did not even get sick despite being deliberately exposed to the virus.

> *Pay attention to your emotional state the next time you become ill. If something has been bothering you, take deliberate steps to feel better (see Process Section) and see if your recovery is faster.*

Other researchers have found that our immune system responds almost instantaneously to our mood/emotional stance. By measuring the immune system using blood samples, they have determined that positive emotions give the immune system a boost while negative emotions diminish it.

Pain

Find a place inside where there's joy, and the joy will burn out the pain.

Joseph Campbell

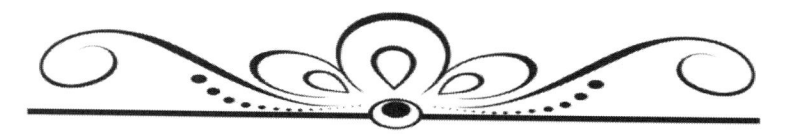

Many people do not want to hear that pain and stress are linked because it reminds them of the older view that pain without a known cause was all in their heads. In one way, that old view was accurate but misunderstood. The pain was because of the perspective the individual took about the situation, which made the person feel stress. They were not imagining the pain. The pain was real.

Individuals who suffer from chronic stress notice the pain is not consistent—it ebbs and flows. Some also notice that it lessens when they feel positive emotion and worsens when they feel negative emotion. Where stress management skills come into play is understanding this connection and using the techniques to create more positive emotions.

Some physicians, such as Dr. John E. Sarno have successfully treated thousands of patients using techniques that recognize the mind-body connection.[39] The success rate of clinical trials conducted on Dr. Sarno's work show statistically significant improvements (54%) in back pain.

The root cause of the pain is physical, but the physical problem is often the result of chronic stress.[40] Our biochemistry changes when we are under stress. The adrenal glands send out adrenaline, cortisol, and other hormones. This response to stress causes the digestive tract to slow down, the heart to beat faster, and muscle tension. In unmanaged chronic stress, the change in biochemistry can lead to physical symptoms including but not limited to heartburn, headache, backache, irritable bowel syndrome, diarrhea, constipation, and more. It can also lead to inflammation and eventually, heart disease. Skin problems, such as psoriasis, are associated with stress.

Chapter 8: Bits and Pieces

OCCUPATION RELATED: NURSES

Your vision of and belief in your ability to become who you want to be is the greatest asset you have.

Unknown

Every occupation has its challenges. In the interest of time and space, I am going to limit my discussion to nurses for a variety of reasons. Much of the discussion about nurses easily transfers to other industries. Nursing, as a rule, has been the subject of more research than many other occupations, which makes it easier to provide a strong foundation for the points that are important to understand in order to increase human thriving.

Nursing is a stressful occupation for many reasons. There are often long hours working in physically challenging conditions. The mental and emotional stress of working with individuals who are ill and making decisions where the consequences can be life threatening is significant. It all adds up and takes a toll. Often, nurses struggle outside of work as well-- in part because their income may have to stretch to cover their expenses and because shift schedules and chronic stress make relationships more difficult to maintain.

Giving nurses training in skills they can use to reduce their own stress levels will increase resilience and emotional intelligence[41], which translates into an easier time for nurses and better nurses for the patients and their employers. Increasing resilience will reduce the likelihood a nurse will decide to leave the profession--something that happens too often and is contributing significantly to the nursing shortage. The nursing shortage, in turn, makes the lives of nurses more difficult because fewer nurses are available to cover multiple shifts. This contributes to longer hours and less flexibility in shifts.

Stress also reduces cognitive function. Reduced cognitive function increases the risk of mistakes.

Then there is the association with pain. Pain is not in one's head, but during low emotional states, the body communicates more of the pain to the conscious mind. When someone is in a good mood, the sensation of pain is reduced. Hospitals with critically ill patients noticed that when the football games were on, the request for pain medicine declined. Some have installed ESPN because of these findings. I notice the connection between pain and good moon when I dance. I can dance for hours without my feet hurting, but when I stop dancing and stand still for a moment, they can put me in agony. Because I understand the link between pleasure and pain, I've played with this, deliberately resuming my dancing while my feet were in agony to see what happens. The pain recedes as soon as I begin dancing to a good song. Nurses often have painful foot and back problems. Stress management skills that help them sustain positive moods could help nurses manage the pain.

Our choice of occupation shapes much of our view of the world. In many occupations, the focus is on finding problems and fixing them. Other occupations place an individual in a situation where it is difficult to trust those around them. Both types of occupations can result in undesired outcomes at home. If one is an attorney, looking for problems in contracts or cases, it would be natural to take that same perspective home. Without conscious deliberate work to do otherwise, it is inevitable. Families do not respond well to that approach.[42]

It is possible to adopt one mindset for home and another for work. Physicians, attorney's, law enforcement, dentists, auditors, and others who are focused on problems at work would do themselves tremendous good if they deliberately cultivate a different perspective for their non-work life. I have had some resistance to the idea that we can have different mindsets in different environments. I usually respond by talking about my daughter's little Maltipoo, Angel. Angel has certain rules she follows in our home. When she stays with the grandparents, who are stricter, she has other rules.

POSTTRAUMATIC GROWTH AND RESILIENCE

Why does one individual who endures a negative life event experience post adversarial growth when another who suffers a similar event develops posttraumatic stress disorder (PTSD) or begins a downward spiral? A resilient person bounces back. Someone who has not developed resilience stagnates.[43] The individual's skill at managing her emotional state is the difference).[44]

Stress can damage health and make life less pleasant in many ways—it can also lead to positive growth. The determining factor is not the severity of the problem or the source thereof. The use of positive coping strategies to solve or manage the problem, taking perspective and self-regulation, allows individuals to benefit from stressful experiences. Unmanaged stress, or to which poor coping skills such as blaming others, escapism, and the use of drugs or alcohol to regulate emotions were associated with poorer outcomes.[45]

Barbara L. Fredrickson, Ph. D. states, "Positivity is perhaps the best kept secret of people who, against all odds, keep on bouncing back."[46] In her research, subjects who had more positive mindsets demonstrated greater resilience. The role positivity plays in resilience is significant. According to Fredrickson, "The most pivotal difference, though, between those with and without resilient personality styles was their positivity. It was the secret of their success. It was the mechanism behind their lesser depression and their greater psychological growth. In short, we discovered that resilience and positivity go hand-in hand. Without positivity, there is no rebound."[47]

Positive emotions have demonstrably beneficial effects when present during times of stress."[48]

♥ Jeanine Joy
TRUE Prevention—Optimum Health

Chapter 9: Perception

We have to remember that what we observe is not nature in itself, but nature exposed to our method of questioning.
Werner Heisenberg

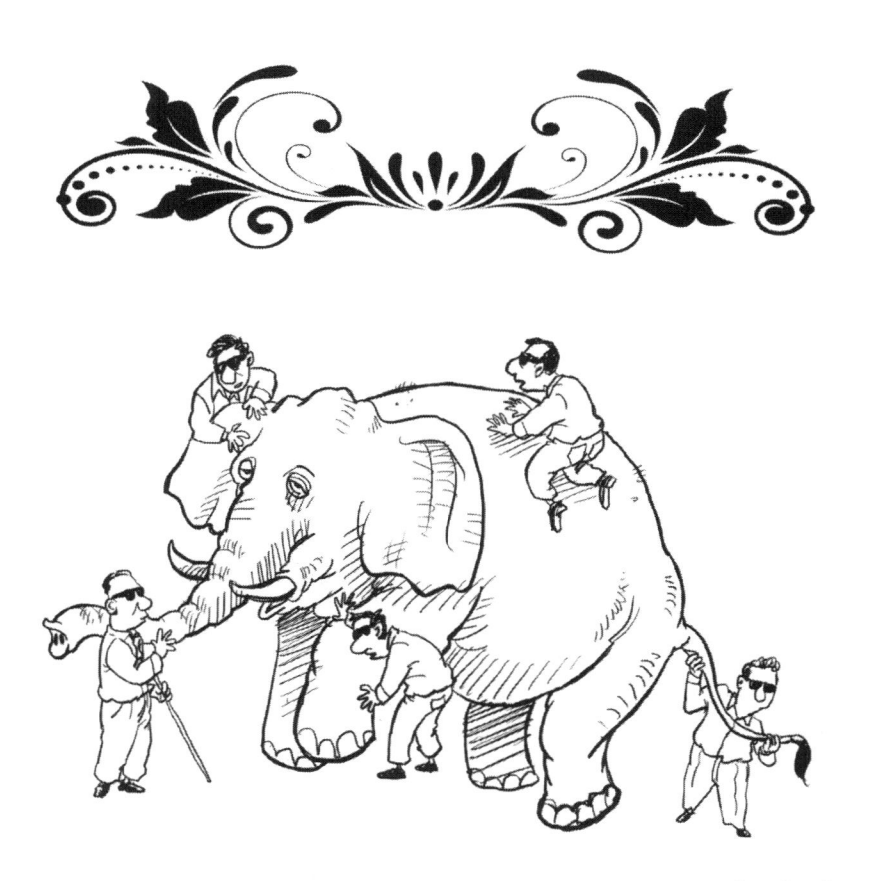

(Dukudraw)

There is a parable that dates back almost a thousand years, with versions in Buddhist, Sufi, Hindu, and Jain lore. You may have heard it elsewhere. It is the story of the five blind men and the elephant.

Once upon a time, there lived five blind men in a village. One day other villagers told them, "There is an elephant in the village today."

They had no idea what an elephant was. They decided, "Even though we will not be able to see it, let us go and feel it anyway." All of them went to the elephant and each touched part of the elephant. One man touched the leg, another touched the tail, a third touched the trunk, one touched an ear, and the final blind man touched the elephant's side.

"The elephant is a pillar," said the first man.
"No! It is like a rope," said the second man.
" No, it is like a thick branch of a tree," said the third man.
"It is like a big hand fan," said the fourth man.
"It is like a huge wall," said the fifth man.

They blind men began to argue about the elephant with each one insisting that he was right. The disagreement was becoming agitated. A wise man was passing by and he saw this. He stopped and asked them, "What is the matter?" They said, "We cannot agree what the elephant is like." Each one of them told what he thought the elephant was like. The wise man calmly explained to them, "All of you are right. The reason every one of you perceives it differently is because each one of you touched different parts of the elephant. The elephant has all those features."

There was no more arguing. The men proceeded to touch other parts of the elephant for themselves, to better understand what their friends had felt.

This parable applies to everyday life far more than most realize. Every aspect of what we perceive as reality—including what we see, smell, taste, touch, and hear—is not only subjective and unique to us, it is also filtered by our beliefs, expectations, emotional stance, and focus. In light of this, disagreements, especially heated ones, become somewhat comical—much like the blind man who felt the tail arguing over the nature of an elephant with the one who touched the ear.

Take a moment and consider how understanding this might influence heated disagreements over social issues, political issues, and religious issues. I'm not foolish enough to dip my toes further in these waters and I believe my readers are intelligent enough to consider that opposing sides simply interpret reality in different ways—not that one is right and one is wrong, but that they are just different.

If the only thing dividing us is based on our personal interpretations of reality, how do we solve such issues? Are they solvable? My recommendation is that the discussions be taken to the deepest level, one where I believe we are all the same. There are only three goals at that level: to love, to be loved, and to leave the world better than we found it. If we focus on the harmony at this level, we will be less insistent that they take the same path to the destination.

Even though this deepest level is not apparent in individuals living in low emotional states, it is there. When their emotional state rises, it can be seen.

Before Chronic Stress is discussed, I am going to introduce several chapters that help the discussion about chronic stress to be deeper and more beneficial to improved health and wellbeing. One of the reasons so many things are not as good as we would like them to be is that the fundamental ways we look at the world are inaccurate. We even know, to some degree, that premises most of us base our opinions and decisions upon are not absolutes, but we do not apply that knowledge to things our senses make us believe are real. It is important that the reader remember that our senses do not *report* reality to us—they *interpret* reality. For some of my readers, this may be an entirely new way of looking at the world. For others, some of it is a refresher course.

There are myriad instances where most adults are aware that what their brains show them about reality is not accurate, but almost no one consciously extends that awareness to a deeper understanding. We often argue and fight with others when both parties are right—each from their own perspective.

Arguments about colors, tastes, sounds, and even intentions, actions, and words cannot be about the actual color, taste, sound, intentions, actions or words because we are not able to perceive any of those things in the exact way another person perceives them. For example, someone who believes the world is good interprets words and actions differently than someone who believes the world is full of evil. We believe we perceive actual reality, but we are not. What we perceive with our eyes, ears, nose, taste[49], and touch are perceived using senses that are not identical to the sensors others' use. Once stimuli is sensed, it goes through a filtering process that distorts our perception in significant ways.

Before arguing with someone, ask yourself if it is possible that each of you is right based on the way you interpret reality.

We attempt to get others to agree with our perspective on something—such as the color of a sofa—when the actual color is a perception that is subjective and greatly influenced not only by the physical apparatus we call a body, but also by our cultural indoctrination. In some cultures, the color wheel is defined differently. In those cultures, the perception of a color is viewed differently than it is in the USA. For example, another culture may consider what I call purple to be blue. When I look at a color, the actual shade, what I see may be different from the shade you see, because of physical differences in our eyes/cones/rods, how we learned to define colors as a child, and because the lighting is different. Even if we are both in the same room at the same time, it is not possible for both of us to have exactly the same angle looking at something as the other has. If we take a picture so we can look at something with the same angle and lighting, the lighting we have when we look at the picture will have the same limitation—we cannot both look at the photograph from the exact same angle in the exact same room at exactly the same time.

Our brains will see something one way, even when we know it can also be viewed another way; the brain is hard pressed to see it both ways at the same time. Life is a combination of events and experiences that pass through filters (which you can control) and comes out on the other side as your emotional experience of the event.

Some people immediately see two faces when they look at the illustration. Others see a vase or goblet. Years ago, when I first saw this illustration, I saw only the vase. It took me a long time to figure out the two faces. I have learned to toggle between seeing the faces and the vase, but I have not been able to see both simultaneously. I can change perspective quickly, but not fast enough that I perceive it as seeing both in the same instant.

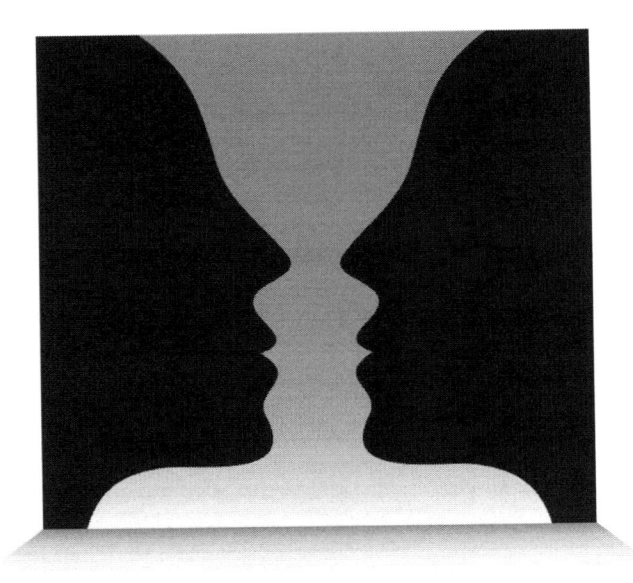

Most of us accept that things referred to as optical illusions trick our minds into seeing something different from what is there, but expanding that concept to understanding what we see is not what is actually there can be a stretch. Our senses are designed to make us believe what we sense is reality. Grasping the concept that it is merely an interpretation is critical to the ability to increase thriving to optimum levels in every area of life.

Once you realize that your opinions, perspective, and beliefs about anything are merely one of many possible accurate interpretations of reality, differences can become interesting instead of points of contention. The conversation changes to one where understanding of the basis of the others' viewpoint is sought, rather than an argument over which an individual is perceiving the situation accurately. As the conversations evolve, there is greater personal discovery about how we perceive the world. Appreciation for our differences increases because it becomes apparent that one perspective is better at solving some issues while another perspective is better at other issues.

We want different things because we have different perspectives. If everyone wanted the same thing, there would be one individual who was the perfect spouse, one perfect job, one perfect physical location to live, and so on. If everyone wanted the same things, everyone except the one who had them would have to settle for less than he desired. We do not have a perfect world, but many people like their mates, jobs, and homes better than those that other people possess.

If all people wanted the same things, the creativity that is so abundant in our world would not have an outlet. Everyone would want the same picture on their walls, the same color houses, and everyone would wear the same clothes. Are you bored yet?

Our unique perspectives create unique desires. Our lack of understanding that others do not perceive reality in the same way we do creates conflicts that are completely avoidable when we make an effort to be more conscious that our perception of reality is individualized.

Optical illusions may only be a cool phenomenon when viewed as something that tricks the mind. Considered from the perspective of "Is my mind showing me an actual reality?" the illusion gains greater meaning and provides insights surface thinking does not begin to consider.

What we perceive is based on so many personal factors. In truth, no two individuals experience exactly the same reality. We are each creating our own version of reality from the information (mainly wavelengths) that exists.

Let's address that for a moment. Human sight is wavelengths in the perceptible range for humans interpreted by the physical apparatus we call eyes and then by the central nervous system and cognitive function of the individual.

We are tricked into believing that reality is an absolute—but reality is an interpretation of wavelengths. Sight is interpretation of wavelengths and sound is also interpretation of wavelengths.

> *Most of our assumptions have outlived their uselessness.*
> **Marshall McLuhan**

If you went through school a while ago, you may remember a map of the tongue depicting where we would taste sweet, salty, bitter, etc. I remember the map not making any sense to me because it did not match my personal experience. In recent years, the research into taste has expanded the reality of how taste is perceived. They have learned that our mood affects taste, what our mothers ate while we were in the womb affects what we like, as does the room we are eating in, and the plates we are eating on. Taste is a combination of input from our tongue, the back of our nose, and even our intestines[50].

Personal biases filter the taste experience in much the same way they filter the information our conscious mind receives in other area. Even what we hear affects how our food tastes—such as crunchy. Our brain takes the inputs and revises them, sometimes beyond recognition.

Our brain combines the information from our senses and determines whether we like the taste. Our brain is also what sees. An individual can experience a brain illness or injury and lose the ability to see in color while the eyes remain perfectly healthy[51].

Chapter 9: Perception

Machinery has enabled us to measure sounds that we cannot hear although we knew there were sounds we could not hear since the time dogs were domesticated. Most of us know dogs can hear things we cannot hear and smell things we cannot smell (thank goodness!). Birds are able to distinguish colors human cannot differentiate. We interpret them as the same as one another, while birds can tell the difference between the two.

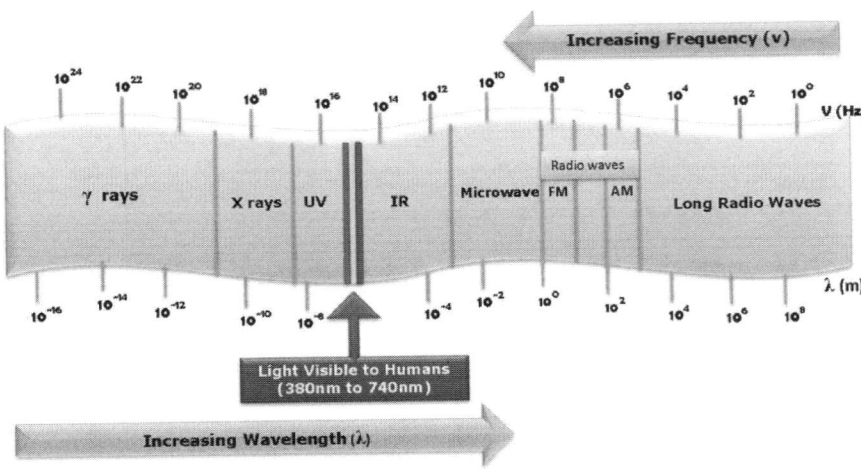

We refer to the wavelengths humans can see as the visual light region but it would be more appropriate to refer to it as the visible by humans light region.

Many things we know about are not explicable using what we know. For example, the cuckoo bird is a brood predator. An avian brood predator lays its eggs in the nest of a host bird that cares for the hatchling. Cuckoo birds are not raised by birds of their species, yet all the fledglings know to migrate and where to go when they migrate. Migration has been explained by "instinct." What is instinct? How does the bird know when to go and where to go? The young birds leave after the adult birds. The round trip from the UK to Africa is 10,000 miles[52]. Instinct appears to be a catch-all phrase used to explain otherwise inexplicable behavior in the animal world. The moth burning itself to death on the hot light seems to meet the definition of predetermined responses to stimuli. More complex behaviors do not fit as neatly.

Is it time to reevaluate instinct based on the Parsimony Principle? The more we learn about non-human behavior, the further the concept of instinct is stretched.

It is not limited to the animal world, however. Every 4th generation of Monarch butterflies migrates to Mexico or California for the winter. Generations 1, 2, and 3 live much shorter lives. Since they cannot survive the climate in most of North America during the colder winter months, the 4th generation flies to warmer climates, ensuring the continuation of the species[53]. How does a butterfly, whose entire body weighs about 2 ounces, know to migrate to Mexico for the winter?

What exactly is instinct? Hundreds of species exhibit behavior we cannot explain any other way. Is it possible they receive some sort of communication or guidance that we cannot detect that directs their actions? It is not blind adherence to something predetermined. Recently, researchers tracking Cuckoo birds noted that birds sometimes return to the last place they were able to forage successfully for food when drought or excessive wetness made food scarce on their usual migration pattern[54].

If they are blindly following instinct, which is what it seems moths do when drawn to a hot light source, how do they vary their behavior when conditions are not favorable for the usual route?

Each of us is essentially hypnotized about the nature of reality from infancy. Cultural anthropologists have thoroughly documented how persons who grow up in different cultures perceive literally different realities[55]. Upon what premises is our "official" concept of reality based? How was that concept determined?

The "Physical Level" of reality is not a static fact. In 1847, when E. Semmelweis suggested physicians should wash their hands between patients and between touching patients and cadavers, he was ridiculed and ignored. Why? Because the "physical world" was not defined in a way that included germs and viruses. Fifty years later, after the invention of the microscope, the definition of our physical reality shifted to include germs, viruses, and other microorganisms that were unknown when the physical world was more narrowly defined. Scientists today, especially quantum physicists, would be quick to confirm the existence of matter and processes we cannot yet measure or define at a physical level. We know of their existence only because the affect they have on things we can measure has been detected and measured.

> *Until you make the unconscious conscious, it will direct your life and you will call it fate.*
>
> *C. G. Jung*

In 1847, Semmelweis demonstrated that the death rate from childbed fever could be reduced from 32% to 1% by introducing the process of hand washing with his patients. Because the world did not understand why hand washing mattered, despite results demonstrating a dramatic difference in the death rate of young women, his recommendation was ridiculed. This is not a human behavior pattern limited to the uneducated masses of earlier times.

Today, there are several areas where our ability to measure our environment has increased. As a result, our understanding of how things are connected is expanding, which is changing individual opinions about some previously controversial topics.

For example, homeopathy has often ridiculed as a hoax, but thousands swear it has helped heal them. Homeopathy involves diluting substances until there was no measurable[1] evidence of the substance. People did not understand how helped because, based on our ability to measure the presence of beneficial substances, no beneficial substances remained in the solution.

Last year, new research demonstrated that classically prepared ultradilute homeopathic medicines (HM) contain measurable source nanoparticle (NP) and/or silica NP with absorbed source materials that are heterogeneously dispersed in colloidal solution and have biological properties that differ substantially from bulk forms of the same substance[5,6]. Our ability to measure nanoparticles expanded, allowing us to physically measure something we previously said did not exist. The view held by many was based on our interpretation of reality, not reality itself.

This is another instance where society's views on a subject have been limited by our ability to take physical measurements. If we could not measure it, we proceed as if it could not exist. Now that the nanoparticles are measurable, it will be interesting to observe the shifts in public opinion about the practice. Homeopathy may begin moving into the mainstream with other Complementary and Alternative Medicines (CAM).

I am not arguing for homeopathy (or against it). I am arguing for minds open enough to consider the possibility that something we do not fully understand (mechanically) but for which there is evidence of a beneficial effect not be dismissed merely because we have not yet learned how or why it works.

Many have argued that the beneficial effect of homeopathy is the placebo effect. I wonder, if in some of the clinical trials conducted, if the nocebo effect might have affected the results. If the clinician conducting the trial did not believe homeopathy was beneficial, her belief could have created a nocebo effect that negated the benefits. I am not stating this is the case, but until it is ruled out, I question the validity of the trials that did not control for this potential.

In many areas of medicine, many relevant factors are considered when we conduct clinical trials, but the mind-body connection is often ignored. The evidence that our immune system functions better when we are positively focused has been demonstrated biologically and in overall health results countless times. Ignoring emotional stance in clinical trials negates the value of the results.

Today we have strong evidence that positivity and optimism reduce the risk of developing heart (cardiovascular) disease by 50%—the number one cause of death in the world—and the advice to increase positivity is mocked and ignored. I have termed this the Galileo Effect—the tendencies to cling to what we already believe regardless of how convoluted our explanations have to become as new information that contradicts the original hypothesis accumulates.

We have ignored the Placebo and Nocebo effect for decades despite the Placebo effect often demonstrating an efficacy rate equal to that of drugs. We have ignored the stunning results from some of the Nocebo trials that have been done. It is common practice for physicians to warn patients about the health problems they are "likely" to experience now that they are X old with no consideration given to the potential nocebo effect from an authority figure advising them they are at risk of experiencing a specific malady. Requests to refrain from providing the warnings are met with statements that the physician's E & O insurance requires him to provide the warnings.

The reality we can ascertain with our physical sensory feedback systems reflects one reality (and not the same one to each of us). The reality we can ascertain with our current technology and measuring capabilities reflects more information than our physical senses communicate to us. I find it impossible to believe that we have reached a stage where we are able to identify and measure everything that is reality. We simply define as reality what we perceive as reality.

For example, when I was reading about the Cuckoo birds, it stated that the males and females of one subspecies were identical in appearance. Many birds are able to distinguish colors that humans cannot perceive with our eyes. Would it not be more accurate to say that Cuckoo's color differentiation, if it exists, is not perceivable by the human eye? Given the amazing and colorful foliage in the animal kingdom, I find it far more plausible that we simply are unable to see the differences not that they do not exist. The Cuckoos may be able to easily discern the difference because their eyes do not have the same specifications as human eyes. Although the research indicating birds can discern differences in bird coloring that humans do not differentiate did not mention Cuckoo birds, there is no reason to believe they cannot until they are studied.

Color is created by our perceptual system, the experience of what we call color is an arbitrary one. Color, pitch, smell, hearing, and taste[57] are all created internally—which explains why some people like a particular smell and others do not[58].

It can be helpful to think of your body as separate from yourself, sort of like a vehicle you operate, limited in what and how it perceives by the installed equipment. If back-up sensors are installed, there is one experience. If a back-up camera is standard equipment, there is another experience. If it has gauges, the experience is different from the experience in a vehicle that only has warning lights. Add a moon roof and the experiences changes even more. A Ford Taurus and a Cadillac Escalade do not get the same gas mileage, the view out the windows is not identical, the sounds perceived within their confines differ from one another.

Our eyes are designed to see between 380 – 740 nanometers, not higher or lower. They interpret the environment within the confines of the specs. Humans do come with different specifications. We are not all identical in our ability to perceive. Some of us have three cones in our optical system and others have four cones. Our ears do the same, hearing within the limited frequency range they are designed to perceive. Bats and dogs definitely hear sounds we do not hear—we do not doubt that they are hearing. We do not tell them they are crazy, making things up, or hearing voices. Following the vehicle analogy, we understand that the vehicles they are utilizing have different specifications than ours.

We also have an onboard computer that checks incoming data against several factors, providing us only with the data it believes is relevant based on its programming. This onboard computer can help us thrive if it is programmed correctly. If the programming is based on unsupportive data—it can make life much more difficult.

If we do not believe something is possible, our brains will not pass on data demonstrating that thing. It will file it in an irrelevant file. If we later decide to believe something different, we can retrieve data from the irrelevant file and evaluate it from a new perspective. An example of this is when someone's spouse cheats but they did not believe the person was capable of doing so. After the fact, the person will often beat themselves up for "not seeing the signs." Understanding that their own brain filed the signs in the irrelevant file because they did not believe their spouse capable of cheating might help them stop the unproductive self-criticism. An individual who does not believe their spouse capable of infidelity has programmed their filters to ignore the warning signs. Signs that might be seen if the spouse was considered capable of infidelity are misinterpreted.

If we expect to have a frustrating encounter, we will interpret the encounter in that way. Have you ever seen someone somewhat upset attempt to solve a problem—perhaps with a front desk person at a hotel? The front desk person can be doing an excellent job, understanding the issue and attempting to provide what most would consider a reasonable solution, but the person who expected to be frustrated does not understand the solution being offered—not because it is complicated, but because their brain is interpreting the situation as expected—frustrating.

If we are chronically appreciative, we will find something to appreciate in even unpleasant circumstances. Our minds evaluate how we the majority of the time and feed us thoughts that are in line with that emotional stance. This is one of the main reasons there are so many individual and unique responses to stimuli.

If you are focused on something, orange cars for example, y your mind will make you more conscious of orange cars. It is not that there are more orange cars; it is that once you program your mind to focus on them, the information is passed to your conscious mind. This filter can be a tremendous tool, when used correctly.

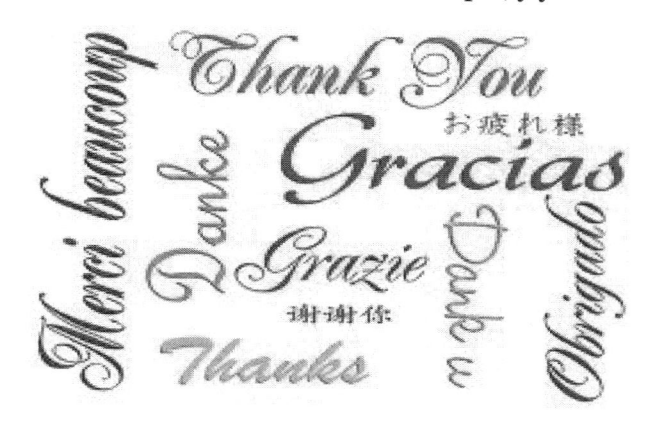

Our vehicles (bodies) are equipped with sensory systems that provide feedback to guide us toward self-realization. We do not have all the options. We cannot see x-rays, we cannot see gamma rays, and we cannot see radio waves. Our vehicles are not equipped with the sensors for those. That does not mean those things do not exist—it simply means we cannot perceive them.

The next few chapters will provide background information about a newly discovered sensory feedback system. (Sensory feedback system is a scientific term that could also apply to our eyes, ears, etc.) This system is called our Emotional Guidance Sensory Feedback System (EGS). One of the reasons our EGS was overlooked in the past is because we have all been taught to misinterpret its signals. The system provides the feedback, but when we misinterpret the meaning, we do not derive the full benefit. Some of the feedback is so natural, and so intuitive, we do not realize what it is. We have had guidance in response to every thought we have thought since birth (or before). It feels natural. A filter I do not often speak about as often is the shift or change filter. This filter highlights new information. It is the reason someone will notice that someone had their hair cut, nails done, lost weight, gained weight, or any number of other changes. The Change/shift filter highlights information that is different. Because our EGS has always been present, we have not noticed it. We have to consciously notice it in order to thrive. Once we understand how it works and make an effort to notice the feedback, it is unmistakable.

A change of perception changes everything. Each mind interprets the world according to factors specific to the individual[59]. These factors create a filtering system in the brain that determines the sensory input that is communicated to the conscious mind. The filtering processes uses the programming of the filters when it determines how we will interpret what we see and experience in the world. When one changes her thoughts, her world changes. People give thoughts power when they accept them as true. Everyone has a choice. Right Responses involve deliberately changing beliefs, expectations, and focus, which results in a different emotional response from our emotional feedback system.

Humanity being taught to misinterpret sensory feedback that is so critical to human thriving was not a deliberate act or intended to cause harm. At least not by those who taught us—the origins are unknown. Misinterpretation has been going on throughout recorded history.

In *Happiness*, Matthieu Ricard[60] writes:

> *"As influential as external conditions may be, suffering, like well-being, is essentially an interior state."*

The amount of stress we feel in any given situation is the direct result of how we perceive that stress[61]. Do we think it is more than we can handle? Do we think we're capable of handling it? Do we see it as specific to this situation or as part of a widespread problem? Have we successfully dealt with this type of situation in the past? Has someone we know or have heard about successfully (or unsuccessfully) dealt with the same problem? The answers we give to these questions and more determine how we experience the moment—including how our bodies respond.

Right now the course of human history is going to change. We, and future generations, will enjoy a kinder[62] and more harmonious world, one where each individual has greater resources than ever before to fulfill his or her own potential. It does not matter who the person is, rich or poor, blue, green, purple, or fuchsia, none of the arbitrary labels that we have used to disempower ourselves, or that others have invoked and convinced us could hold us back, will hold anyone back unless they allow them to do so. The truth is, it has always been this way, but without understanding our guidance to help overcome adversity, almost no one could find the path. Now it is a bright line for anyone who takes the time to learn these skills.

Chapter 10: Intro to Emotional Guidance

No man can reveal to you aught but that which already lies half-asleep in the dawning of your knowledge.
The teacher who walks in the shadow of the temple, among his followers, gives not of his wisdom but rather of his faith and his lovingness.
If he is indeed wise he does not bid you enter the house of his wisdom, but rather leads you to the threshold of your own mind.
Kahlil Gibran

It is time for you to learn how to interpret your Emotional Guidance System (EGS) accurately. As your understanding grows, you will become aware of more and more subtleties, the awareness of which makes your life feel easier and easier. Beneficial synchronicities will begin to show up in your experiences.

Our emotions are actually a sensory feedback system designed to guide us to self-realization. Self-realization, as intended here, refers to movement toward the full development of one's abilities and talents. It is toward, rather than the fulfillment of, because as we achieve more, our ability to continue to achieve expands—there is no end to what can be accomplished by an individual who continually moves in the direction of self-realization.

There are many ways to explain how our emotions work to provide us with guidance. Subsequent chapters will explore some of the science supporting this newly recognized sensory feedback system.

Before delving into the science and some of the very practical applications of the guidance, a foundation of the basics of how to use the guidance is needed. When fully understood, the guidance our emotions provide is simple enough for anyone, even children, to use to enhance their life experiences.

I hope you find this chapter fun. I'm going to utilize a different method to introduce the basics of our emotional guidance system. Because using one's emotional guidance is largely a mental process, a topic that can

Chapter 10: Intro to Emotional Guidance

be quite boring to describe in a non-fiction book, I wrote a non-fiction book in which the main character teaches this process. I use an excerpt from that book to introduce the basic premise.

You need some background on the characters to understand the scene. The main character, Maia, teaches human thriving in our time. She has been transported to the future, a world divided into a Utopian society filled with individuals who understand their emotional guidance, and a Dystopian society filled with violence, shorter life spans, and other undesirable traits. The geo-political map in this future time bears little resemblance to what we know today. The Dystopian society is divided into territories led by violent, dictator-like warlords.

The Utopian society (Solis) brought Maia to the future, but she has now been kidnapped by Marcello, the leader of the largest Dystopian territory. I hope you enjoy this excerpt from Shades of Joy:[63]

Marcello led Maia to a cozy library," Will this be an acceptable classroom?"

Maia looked around the room filled with rich cherry cabinets climbing high up the tall ceilings; a ladder was needed to reach the top shelves. She was delighted to see some classics on the shelves. Her heart was gladdened to know the book burning had not been as thorough as she had feared. There was a fireplace flanked by large windows that looked out onto Puget Sound. Two comfortable chairs were situated in front of the unlit fireplace and Turkish rugs graced the hardwood floors.

"Yes, this will do. Do you have a white board?"

"A white board?"

"Yes, a board where I can sketch out concepts to make them easier to understand."

"I don't have one. I will have one of my men check on it. Couldn't we just use paper?"

"Paper will do for now." Maia stated, "But a white board would be helpful as we move along."

Maia sat in the chair to the left and waited for Marcello to sit in the other.

"The first thing you have to understand is the path to where you want to go is the path to happiness. I will speak often of happiness. I don't know how happiness is viewed here. It would help if you shared that with me."

"Happiness?" Marcello laughed harshly, "Happiness is a myth."

Maia took a deep breath. "I assure you, happiness is not a myth. It is a reality for many people and attainable by all. It is the primary motivation for everything you have ever done."

"Bah! You don't know anything about why I do what I do."

"I know far more than you believe and more than you do, I am sure. By the end of our time together, you will understand how that is true. However, you have a decision to make. One I thought we covered this morning. Do you want to learn my secrets, or do you want to argue with me?"

"How could you know more about my life than I do?" Marcello visibly bristled at Maia's words.

Maia could tell it was all bluster. Marcello had been behaving that way so long; he no longer even realized it was not the way he wanted to behave. Should she kowtow to him or stay in her power? That was a silly question. She was an indomitable force when she stayed in her power. He would not harm her as long as she had the secrets to what he wanted. Once he had the secrets, he would no longer want to harm her.

"Do you want to remain ignorant of the truth? Right now, you know so little about the truth that you cannot understand or comprehend it when you hear it. I know the secrets to a life that is as good as one can be. I know that is something you could have. But, more importantly, all the people in your territory could have better lives."

She paused and felt greatly rewarded when she saw a spark of interest in Marcello's eyes following her last statement. "I am happy to teach you what I know, but you have to be the student. In time, we will learn from one another. However, your only job right now is to let me know whether you understand what I say. You must keep an open mind, or you will not hear or understand."

Marcello sighed while visibly relaxing. "I want to learn, but you make no sense."

"The reason I make no sense is because you have been lied to your entire life; this entire society is full of lies—lies and false premises that lead everyone astray."

"My father did not lie to me."

"I am not saying he lied intentionally." Maia realized the beginning would be a slow start. "He was lied to, and his Father before him, and so on back through time."

Brushing a stray hair away from her face Maia said, "Let me begin again."

"There are things about your brain that few people understand. Let me explain those things, and we may be able to move more quickly once that understanding exists. What do you believe the function of your brain is?"

"It is for rational, unemotional thought. It is to give me information to make good decisions, for remembering and on an unconscious level, it beats my heart, keeps me breathing when I sleep, and more."

"Those are pretty common beliefs, but they are not accurate. Before we are done you will see that what you considered 'rational thought' is actually the most irrational thoughts you have access to." Seeing Marcello about to protest once again, Maia stated, "Don't interrupt."

Maia calmly watched his face; rage was his first response to her insolent comment. Soon, he gained control of the rage and overrode it with his desire to understand what she knew. Maia waited until his face showed he was receptive to her words before continuing. "Your brain's primary job is to prove your own beliefs to you. It filters out information that contradicts your beliefs, and perceives information in a way that is consistent with your existing beliefs. It does not care if your beliefs are true, or if they serve you. It only cares if the information is presented in a way that is consistent with your established beliefs."

Pausing to allow Marcello time to absorb the enormity of her comment, Maia continued. "It is easier to see it in others than in ourselves. Think for a minute about people you know. Maybe someone who believes they are not treated fairly, but you believe they are. How do they perceive life? Do they perceive it as if life is unfair to them?"

Maia could see Marcello considering her words. She decided she needed to move slowly through this initial stage until he trusted her.

"Think about it for a few minutes. Look for examples of people who believe life is a certain way and make excuses for why others' lives are different from their own."

Maia rose and went to a bookshelf where she had spotted a book of quotes. Unsure of what she might find within its pages, but hopeful, she returned to her seat with the heavy book. Paging through she found the category 'Expectation' and scanned the quotes. Grinning when she found the one she sought, she said, "I like to share the wisdom of the ages with my students. This wisdom has been known throughout history. "I have just put all the pieces together in a way that provides answers and helps humans thrive. That is what is unique about my methods—I have connected more dots than others." Looking back at the book, she read, 'Whether you believe you can, or you believe you can't, either' Marcello joined her as she said the last words, 'way you're right. Which are you? Henry Ford.'"

"How did you know I love that quote?"

"I didn't. It is a favorite of mine as well. Without my usual resources available, I have to improvise with what is available. I will tell you something else you will not yet understand: I was guided to use it."

"Don't lie to me! There is no one else here. You were not guided. Don't give me your superstitious mumbo jumbo. I want clear answers."

"Marcello," Maia said with a calm voice while reaching out and touching his arm, knowing the Reiki energy would help calm not only his temper, but also his wounded spirit. "No one is alone in this life. We can choose to feel alone. We can choose to act alone. Nevertheless, all of us have guidance that is available to us in every moment. At any time, we are free to tune in to it and use its power to aid us. Have you never known to do, or not do, something but not known why? Known it so strongly that nothing could convince you otherwise? When you know that strongly, aren't you always right?"

Maia saw the recognition of unexplained knowledge in his eyes.

"It's not there all the time." He said. "Usually, I don't know. But sometimes, yes, there have been times when I knew without knowing how I knew. Bringing you here was one of those times."

"Then do not waste the opportunity by arguing with everything I say. Clearly, your guidance is telling you I have something you want very badly. When someone is not usually tuned to their guidance, they still notice it when the urges are powerful. Once again, may I have your agreement—this time I want your word on it—that you will stop arguing with me?"

Maia thrust her right hand toward Marcello. She was not sure if a handshake still had the meaning attributed to it in her time but she was willing to hope.

Marcello eyed her warily, dismayed by her offer. She waited, leaving her hand outstretched while he decided. She could see the resignation in his eyes as he clasped hers and shook.

"Good. Now that that's out of the way, do you see how Henry Ford's quote is saying much of what I said? Our belief, or expectation, impacts the outcome."

"Yes, and I've seen it in my men as well."

"Thank you. A straight-forward answer." Maia smiled sweetly. "Did you understand that their brains actually filter out solutions, when they don't believe they can accomplish something, and help them find them, when they believe they can?"

"No, I did not make that correlation. So, if I believe something, my brain provides evidence to prove it to me? It interprets reality differently than it would if my beliefs were different?"

"Exactly! You've got it. That is step one. The next step is to begin recognizing when it happens, to you and others. A couple of keys are to recognize, in yourself, when you believe something is true for you but not for others. Remember, beliefs are able to help or hinder. They are not all good or all bad. Most importantly, the brain does not differentiate between those that serve our higher good, and those that thwart it. It 'irrationally' attempts to support whatever we have decided to believe."

"A couple of things may help you identify beliefs that are not serving you. If you find yourself saying, 'I want to but,' you are pointing out a belief that limits you. The second is when you believe that another has it better than you, and have an excuse or explanation for why that is. Think about that for a bit while I think about the best next step."

Marcello looked steadily into Maia's eyes after a few minutes of looking out the window with his eyes brows furrowed, he said, "Do you realize you have already shattered a paradigm I have lived with my entire life?"

"Yes, I do." Maia laughed. "Get used to it. I am going to do it again, but first, there is something you need to know. You can't go back. What I teach, you cannot unlearn. Your worldview will change. We are not so far down the path now that you cannot stop, but soon much of what you have believed will lie in shreds on the floor. I can lead you in a way where you feel good about that, instead of bad that you lived so long with misleading beliefs, but you have to trust me if we are to move forward."

"If I can't trust my brain, what may I trust?"

"Your Emotional Guidance System. I will call it your EGS for short."

"Trust a woman to tell me to trust my emotions!"

"Marcello, emotions are far more valuable and accurate than you understand. It is not the inaccuracy of emotions, but humanity's lack of understanding of the language they use, that makes them seem irrational. I will teach you to understand them. Once you do that, they will never again seem irrational. Let me give you an example. Did your men relay to you anything about my behavior after they kidnapped me? Anything that seemed unusual or unexpected to you?"

"Yes, they wondered if you were crazy. You did not seem docile, yet you came with them almost willingly after the initial confrontation. Yet, you also did not seem afraid to speak up or let them know that something was unacceptable to you."

"Do you have any idea why that might be? How could a woman grabbed in the middle of the night by two men, one of them as big as a mountain with a deformed face that helped to hide the kindness in his heart, not be deathly afraid?"

Marcello shook his head. He had wondered about it. He even, briefly, considered if this was all a set-up, if Maia was a spy. However, Brazil was too far away to impact his territory so that hadn't made sense.

"Tell me."

"After the initial shock, I checked in with my EGS. I understand its language. I also know that at low emotional states my thinking is impaired, and the better-feeling my current emotional stance, the better my cognitive abilities. At first, I wanted to assuage my fears so that I could think of a way to escape. I am not accustomed to feeling bad-feeling emotions. I have mastered techniques that allow me to self-manage myself into consistently good-feeling emotional states most of the time and to, at a minimum, know I am able to return to feeling good in short order if something goes poorly."

"What is 'emotional stance'?"

"There are two ways I will use the term. One is the emotional stance in any given moment—how an individual feels in that single space in time. The other is their chronic emotional stance. Both impact behavior and how the world is perceived. I will tell you more about that later."

"Right now I want to make a different point." Maia gently led him back to discussing her reaction to being kidnapped, feeling they were on the brink of his understanding an important concept more fully.

"One way to feel better when something feels bad is to go more general. I could not come up with a specific plan for escape, especially the further they took me from Solis. Racking my brain for the specifics felt worse. But, I could go general and find thoughts that soothed my fears. I thought things like, "I don't have to figure this out right now." and "I will find a way. " Since I understand how accurate my EGS is, because I habitually use it in my life, when I felt better not only did I feel better, but I knew those statements were true."

"The only way to know with certainty that things that feel better are true is to use your EGS frequently, beginning with small things that are easy to verify. As your trust in your guidance builds, you will begin using it on bigger things. I am considered very rational and analytical. At first, I used both my emotional guidance and my 'rational brain' on a subject. In time, I came to rely less on my 'rational brain' and far more on my EGS. My life has gotten continually better as a result."

Marcello laughed, "You want me to believe your life has gotten continually better yet here you sit, kidnapped, at my mercy." His laugh grew in volume until his entire body shook with his amusement.

Maia sat serenely in her chair, not bothered at all by his finding humor in her statement. "Au contraire, I began this day taking a boat ride, on a dazzling sunny day, across Puget Sound in the most luxurious yacht I have had the pleasure of boarding. My ride was enhanced by a spectacular view of Mt. Rainier. I was given a delicious meal that I did not have to purchase or prepare, ate it at a table with a resplendent view of the sound and of a very attractive man. Then I enjoyed a period of rest where I bathed in luxury and saw a bathtub that I will be able to enjoy later. I am savoring the anticipation of it now. My biggest passion in life is helping others thrive more. Even though you are one of the most powerful men in the world, you are not, and have not been, thriving. Your life is killing you inside. You brought me here to heal that. The potential for good to come from this situation, good that is in alignment with my ultimate desires, is tremendous. Now I sit with an intelligent man who wants to learn what I know in one of the most magnificent libraries that I have ever had the pleasure of enjoying. The Biltmore is more impressive, but this is lovely and I will not diminish it by wishing myself elsewhere. My guidance assures me I am not in danger."

With fiery conviction in her eyes, Maia met Marcello's gaze, defying him to see her reality in a less favorable light. They locked gazes, her conviction firm until Marcello gave her the point, "Touché."

Then he looked down and shook his head. "I see I have a powerful adversary."

"No, you do not. I am not your adversary. At least not in my book. You want to learn what I know. I want you to understand what I know. I know what will happen when you know it. That is the only advantage I have."

"How are you so sure you're not in danger?"

"I have been using my guidance for years. It tells me, loudly, when there is danger and helps me avert or avoid it. When an obstacle in the road ahead while I am driving necessitates a change of lanes, I know before I see the danger. If someone comes to my door that I should not allow inside, it lets me know before I open the door. It works. It knows far more than I have the ability to know through any other means. I trust it implicitly, without exception."

"How can you have such a positive outlook on your situation?"

"I can't have a bad outlook on my situation. Beliefs are just the first filter that distorts the information our rational brain transmits to us. Our habitual emotional stance creates another filter. Because I manage my emotional stance to a place that feels good on a consistent basis, my filter highlights information that feels good to me. It also dims negative aspects."

"But, like I said before, it will tell me of danger. In fact, one of the first ways I learned to trust my EGS was because of what I termed my 'creep alert'. Back then, I was like most of humanity, trained away from my guidance and toward my 'rational mind.' Someone came into my experience and I had a strong and immediate negative reaction to him. I talked myself out of it. Even though I am not a racist person, I told myself that I was being racist. I did not understand the wisdom of one's guidance and thought the only way, or reason, I would have to distrust this individual was because he was a different race than I. I ignored the fact that his first cousin, who was almost twice his size and should have seemed more dangerous, if racism was the reason for my reaction, was someone I was drawn to. In fact, I was enjoying his first cousin's company and developing a friendly, fun relationship that included easy bantering with him."

"My 'rational mind' discarded this evidence and highlighted the fact that I was having this reaction to someone of a different race, for no known reason. My rational mind deduced the reason must be racism. At that time, I did not believe I had guidance. Since I did not have an established belief that I had reliable guidance, my rational mind could not attribute my appropriate response to guidance. It had to supply some other reason for my reaction. It was aware of racist individuals in the world. I believed there were racist people in the world. So, my so-called rational mind irrationally attributed that trait to me to explain what it was unable to explain within my existing belief system in another, more accurate way. Not only did my 'rational mind' discount the first cousin, it discounted countless other experiences in my life that clearly demonstrated I'm not racist—events involving the same race that this man was. The man I had the intense negative reaction to robbed us that same night. Conversing with a friend who was also there, and also not a racist individual, based on many experiences we had previously shared, I learned he had the same reaction and had talked himself out of the feelings for the same reasons I had."

"From that experience, I learned that my 'creep alert' as I termed it, was an accurate predictor of undesired behaviors. I did not know why, but I began listening to it. Later, when I learned more about the EGS, it made sense. So, I am able to maintain a positive outlook because I have developed that habit of looking at life. It does not mean I will not know about danger, or take appropriate action. In fact, I have had experiences where my creep alert has let me know about danger and I have been able to take evasive actions. My focus in those situations is far more on appreciation for having my guidance than in seeing the world as an evil place full of trouble."

"Why did it not warn you away from harm last night?"

"I have not been harmed. In fact, as I said a minute ago, this may be the path of least resistance to goals that are important to me. What made me get up in the middle of the night and take a run? It was the first time I had done that, ever. Perhaps my guidance was leading me to a situation that left the least probability that others would be harmed when I was taken. Had you considered that? I have. In fact, I believe that is why I was inspired to go for a run. Do not try to tell me your men would not have harmed anyone who stood in their way. I know they would have done whatever was necessary to follow your order to bring me to you."

"You have that much faith in your guidance?"

"That and more, but I do not expect you to have faith in yours until you practice. You must begin using your guidance to check things, even as you continue to make decisions the same way you always have. It won't be long until you begin seeing how trustworthy your guidance is. Only you can build your own trust in your guidance. It is a three-pronged approach. First, you have to pay attention to it and begin trusting it. As it proves its value to you, you have two jobs. The first is to listen for and check in with the guidance. It has always been there, but how often have you actually listened? Since you did not know you had guidance, you have really only listened when it was screaming at you. The guidance will guide you in every moment, if you listen carefully."

"I don't want something else telling me what to do." Marcello protested.

"What is it guiding you to?" Maia patiently inquired.

"I don't know. But, I am in charge of my life. I make my own decisions about what I want."

Maia relaxed back in the comfortable chair, allowing Marcello to absorb what he had just stated before asking, again, "What does your guidance guide you to?"

"How should I know? I am not even sure I have this guidance. It sounds impossible."

Enjoying herself greatly, but hiding most of her mirth, Maia repeated the question again, "What does your guidance guide you to?"

"Why do you keep asking me that?"

"Because you told me you do not want your guidance telling you where to go. If you do not know what it guides you to, how do you know?"

Deflated, Marcello finally understood he had been making a decision without knowing what he did not know. "What does my guidance want me to do?"

Giving Marcello an encouraging smile, Maia began the explanation, "It guides you to the dreams, goals, and desires that you have decided you want."

"It guides me to my goals? How does it know what my goals are? I don't tell anyone what all my plans are." Marcello protested.

"I can't tell you the mechanics of how it knows. But, you can show yourself that is what it does—in many ways it seems magical. It will take into account goals that seem to conflict and actually guide you to a path where both may be accomplished—but you are able to get there only if you trust it. As long as your 'rational mind' believes you must make a choice between the two, it will not show you the path to achieve both. However, your EGS will. The clearer you are about your goals, the clearer the guidance you receive. You do not have to even know or remember your goals or desires for your guidance to include them. I have been led to outcomes I had forgotten I wanted; only remembering having that desire when it showed up in my life."

"Then how do you know your guidance led you there?"

"It really is much easier to understand as you experience it. I know there is a level of energy below what we can measure, on the level of Quantum Physics. We feel things from that level. The more we pay attention to how things feel, the more sensitive we become to our own guidance. In many ways, guidance is like our other senses. Our eyes interpret light waves that are translated into what we see. Our ears interpret sound waves that we cannot see. We do not doubt our ears—even though we cannot see the sound waves. Our taste buds translate molecules into specific tastes. Our nose translates the vibration of scents we cannot see, enabling us to smell. Do we ask our nose if the smell we enjoy is real? We were trained to trust those senses, so we do not question them. Our emotions are also sensory feedback. We question them only because we were trained to disregard them. We were trained to believe emotions are unreliable and irrational. We were trained that our "rational minds" are the source of intelligent decisions. Most people still believe that. They do not know the real function of the "rational mind" is to prove our own beliefs to us."

Marcello was listening intently. Maia believed much of what she said was resonating with him on a deep level.

"Our 'rational mind' do not consider what is best for us. They trust that we have established beliefs that serve us. Unfortunately, society did not train us to do that. Society trained us to establish beliefs that were similar to those around us. For the most part, beliefs are passed from parent to child with little change. Teachers pass on their beliefs, not realizing that many of the beliefs they share have the opposite effect of what they truly desire—which is helping students live a better life."

"I will give you some practice exercises to help you begin understanding. Sometimes it will seem to be leading you in the wrong direction. I have learned that if I trust my guidance is taking me the right way, it actually knows the quickest path to my goals. Only in hindsight does the route make sense to me. With enough practice, full faith that you are on the path you want to be on is possible—just by paying attention to your EGS. When you get to that point, life becomes incredibly awesome."

"I can't imagine ever trusting it that much." Marcello's doubts were evident.

"Don't worry about it. Trust will come in time. You will be ready when you are ready. But first, you have to understand its language. Let me see if I am able to be succinct in this explanation."

Maia shut her eyes for a moment, concentrating on allowing the best words to flow through her. Laughing, she jumped up and grabbed what looked like a solid gold pen from Marcello's hand. 'Go stand in the corner with your eyes closed."

He looked like he was going to refuse, but the determined look in Maia's eyes seemed to persuad him to do as she requested.

She looked around the room for a place to hide the pen. There was a very large book on a shelf midway through the room. She lifted it up and slid the pen under it. She was glad the room did not need dusting because disturbed dust would have given the hiding spot away. She then continued walking to the far end of the room, slowly, and then back to where Marcello stood in the corner. She wanted him to hear her steps throughout the room so he would not know by the sound of her steps where the pen was hidden.

She touched him on the shoulder and told him, "You may open your eyes and turn around now."

She returned to the chair she had been using. "Your guidance guides you away from danger and toward thriving. I have hidden your pen. I am going to use clues to help you find it. I will tell you, 'You're getting warmer' when you move toward your pen and I will say, 'You're getting colder' when you are moving away from your pen. Got it?"

"Warmer is toward and colder is away?"

"Yes, much like positive emotions are toward and emotions that feel worse are away."

"If emotional guidance is that simple, how could we be so confused?"

"Well, for one thing, most people will interpret fear as meaning that the thought they just thought is true. When in reality, it means that the thought is moving away from their dreams, desires, and goals if the fearful thought felt worse than the thought before it. Someone could be in such an awful place that a fearful thought actually feels better, but that is a lesson for another day."

Widening her stance, Maia playfully put her hands on her hips and ordered, "Stop stalling and find your pen."

Gaping at her before deciding to join in her playfulness, Marcello took a step toward the far end of the library and Maia said, "You're getting warmer."

He moved slowly and deliberately toward the other end of the library with Maia giving a clue after each step. When he had passed the hiding place far enough that it was behind him she said, "You're getting colder."

Marcello turned toward the books lining the wall opposite where the pen was hidden, taking a step toward them. "You're getting colder." Maia said with a giggle, knowing he would soon have his pen back and gain a rudimentary understanding of emotional guidance.

Marcello turned with more assurance toward the opposite wall.

Maia said, "You're getting warmer."

He moved to the wall and she said, "You're getting quite warm."

He had a smile on his face now as he studied the books before him. He reached out and opened a drawer that was hidden, built to look like it was part of the shelf, but there was no pen inside. Maia remained silent. He looked at her and she laughingly said, "Your guidance will be more specific than I am."

His eyes returned to the books in front of him. He removed a book close to the one his pen was hidden under and Maia said, "You're getting hot."

Marcello seemed to think she had hidden it behind the books as he drew out another one, looking behind. Maia said, "Hot, hot, hot! That would equate to interest or passion if it were your EGS letting you know how close to the right path you are on."

Marcello drew out the book the pen was hidden under by sliding it along the shelf and the pen fell, landing on top of his shinny patent leather shoe.

Marcello picked up the pen and said, "What is my prize?"

"Your prize is a greater understanding of your emotional guidance. Most people think when they feel an emotional response to a thought that feels worse, the emotion is a warning, telling them the thought is something to fear, worry, fret about, or feel concern about. That interpretation is off the mark. Just like, 'You're getting colder' means you are moving away from your goal, those emotions are communicating that you are off-track."

"Each thought you think elicits an emotional response. If the thought is much like the prior thought, there will not be much emotional variance in response to the thought. However, if someone is thinking about a loved one and feeling love but then they think about something that could be of concern, they feel an emotional response that feels worse. For example, let's say your daughter is out with friends. You think about her and feel the love you have for her. Then you think about young people driving and you feel fearful for her safety. The emotional response is not saying, 'Yes, that is a valid worry.' The emotional response is saying, 'You're getting colder,' moving away from what you desire. Energy flow follows your attention. Attention to the unwanted increases the probability of the unwanted."

"The layers in that single scenario are deep and complex. You do not create what will happen in your daughter's life, but you have the power of influence. The first thing that happens is within your own body. When you feel positive emotions, your body thrives; it functions at its optimum level. Your immune system works best when you feel positive emotions and much of one's health flows from that. The life expectancy in Solis is far longer than in the dark zones. Cognitive abilities are at their best when one feels positive emotions and decrease as negative emotions increase. So moving from feeling love for your daughter, to worry or fear, decreases your ability to think clearly."

"An individual who is feeling love treats others well. An individual who is worried or fearful is far more likely to snap at another person, be grumpy, or even say hurtful things to a loved one. Relationships are diminished when the parties in the relationship have chronic thoughts that elicit a bad-feeling emotional response."

"There are other repercussions. Racism increases with negative emotion. The ability to negotiate increases with positive emotions. Access to insights and inspirations increases as habitual positive emotions increase."

"Is this beginning to make sense to you?" Maia checked in to see whether Marcello was keeping up.

"It makes sense when you say it. But when I compare it to what I think I know, the differences make it confusing again." He admitted.

"Relax. You will learn better if you relax into this. You have a lifetime of false premises to overcome. You are not going to grasp it all in one day. I didn't understand it all at once. In fact, there were things that were so contrary to what I believed that I skipped them for a while. I just told myself, the rest of this makes so much sense, I am going to learn all I am able to and come back to that idea when I have a better understanding. Now I know that the areas I had the most difficult time were because I had very strong practiced beliefs that contradicted the truth. Once I experimented with the rest of it and began trusting my guidance, I was able to come back to those areas and understand them. I am a very different person than I was before I understood my EGS. I am far wiser, but also kinder, gentler, more serene, confident, and so much more. Who I used to be is a mere shadow compared to who I have become."

Maia's eyes were shining as she spoke of how far she had come on her own journey. "The old me would be fighting like a cornered tigress with cubs at being kidnapped. Some people might think that was the right response. But I know, based on the feedback from my EGS that this is on a path of least resistance to the accomplishment of my goals. If I was fighting, I would not be moving toward my goals. At the same time, my unproductive emotional stance, panic, fear, hatred, would be growing."

"That response would not serve me or my goals. It would have been merely the trained response of a mind conditioned to resist what it did not understand. I achieve more when I pay attention to the subtler clues guidance provides. Does that give you a glimpse of the type of difference understanding ones guidance could make?"

"I think so. I need to think about it."

"Yes, you do. You'll be able to do that soon."

"Before we break, you need to know a little more. To use your EGS, all you have to do is think of a thought, think it, and pay attention to how it feels. Does it feel warmer or colder? In other words, does the emotional response to the thought feel better emotionally or worse emotionally? I try not to refer to emotions as positive or negative, although I do not always succeed. All emotions are good. They are guidance. Our job is to find thoughts that lead to better-feeling emotions."

To emphasize this important point, Maia said, "A road sign that says, 'Danger Ahead' is not a bad sign. In many ways, the sign is good because it gives warning that a different route might serve you better."

Marcello nodded.

"I want you to practice paying attention to your thoughts, and your emotional response to those thoughts until tomorrow afternoon. That is enough for today. It is a lot to absorb. I want to be able to sleep in tomorrow without worrying about what time I need to get up. What is for dinner?"

I hope you enjoyed the excerpt from Shades of Joy and that it helped you understand how emotional guidance works. In the next chapter, the subject of emotional guidance will be covered from a more scientific perspective.

Chapter 11: Emotional Guidance Sensory Feedback System (EGS)

Just as your car runs more smoothly and requires less energy to go faster and farther when the wheels are in perfect alignment, you perform better when your thoughts, feelings, emotions, goals, and values are in balance.

Brian Tracy

Emotions are the sensory feedback from our oldest sensory system. There is scientific evidence that demonstrates even one-celled organisms have an Emotional guidance System (EGS). Researchers say humans are the only animal that disregards the feedback in favor of the 'rational mind'. The emotional feedback, when understood, provides far better guidance than the rational mind.

The EGS appears to consider information available on the quantum level of physicality. The EGS also appears to bypass the filters that distort information our conscious mind receives from our other senses. The only reason humanity is not thriving is because we have been taught to misinterpret the feedback from our guidance.

The actual job of the rational mind, as you'll learn in the next chapter, is to prove our personal beliefs to us and create meaning from our experiences. This would be fine if the beliefs were deliberately crafted in a society that understands the impact of beliefs and nurtures beliefs that lead to thriving. We do not have that luxury. Many common beliefs diminish thriving yet our rational minds trap us into lives that repeatedly prove those realities to us.

In this chapter, I will provide some of the science behind the emotional sensory feedback system as the scientists refer to it.

As discussed in earlier chapters, the common explanations of ill-health and social problems are complex. That complexity is largely because we have too long held onto a concept that is not true about the origin of both ill health and social ills.

Chapter 11: Emotional Guidance Sensory Feedback System (EGS)

Excessive stress was suggested as a cause of all major disease in 1978. A strong link between stress and cancer was reported in research.[64] A similar relationship between stress and heart disease was suggested in 1981.[65]

At the time, recommendations were made to avoid excessive stress, monitor stress, and remove stressors when possible. For all practical purposes, this advice was useless to most of humanity. Life in the 20th and 21st centuries is stressful for almost everyone. There is so much stress, we have begun building language around the concept: time stress, financial stress, relationship stress, definition of self-stress, socio-economic stress, and stress from wars, fluctuating economies, discrimination, and much more. There is stress from the frequent (and often conflicting) information about what is healthy to eat.

At a time when there were more divorces, blended families, re-evaluation of social and professional roles, redefining of social values, and much more rapid change the level of stress continually increased for most individuals. Stress is much like the old analogy of the boiled frog. The metaphor is that if you put a frog in a pot of water and heat it very gradually, the frog will not jump out and will remain until boiled to death. Whereas if you put him in hot water, he would jump out immediately.

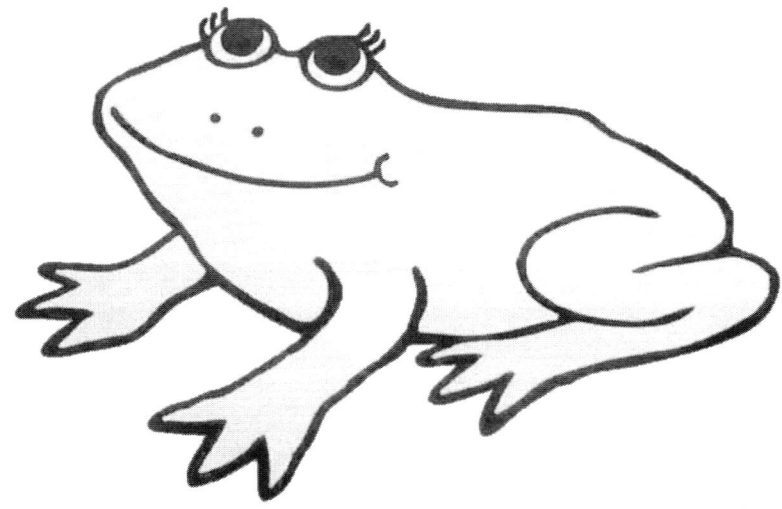

Whether a frog will actually remain in the pot long enough to die is subject to debate. I am not going to try, so we'll leave it as an analogy—a very valid analogy about human behavior.

One of the most common situations where we see this play out is in the area of abusive relationships. This is true of both abused women and men. If the abuser began the relationship with abuse, the abused partner would have left immediately. The abuse would not have been tolerated beyond the first incidence. Abusers tend to introduce abuse gradually, increasing the reign of terror as their victims' tolerance increases. Those watching from the outside have difficulty understanding why the behavior is tolerated.

Abuse is a form of stress. The boiled frog analogy works with employees, too. If the employer had asked for what is demanded a few years into the arrangement on the first day of work, the employee would have immediately looked for a better job. Because demands increase gradually, we do not respond to the increasing levels of stress the same way. We are used to suffering with the level of stress and we continue to accept more until the proverbial straw that breaks the camel's back—which may be in the form of depression, heart disease, divorce (from taking the stress home), cancer[66] or other illness.

It is not all the employer's fault. Employees need to communicate when the demands on them are stretching their ability to deliver. Bosses often forget all an employee's current tasks when more is requested. A long time ago, I worked for one of the big box banks. My schedule was four ten-hour days. One of my peers once remarked, "You don't work 4/10's. You work 7/14's." Unfortunately, she was right. However, the fault was not all on my management. I did not push back. I worked remotely and most of my interaction was across department lines and with other people around the country—not with my boss. My boss probably had no idea how many hours I was putting in.

It is easy to believe that if you push back it will reflect poorly on your performance evaluation. The truth is, the reason you are overloaded is probably because you are reliable. The boss knows that work sent your way is done right the first time. The boss is not overloading you with work because he dislikes you, although you may perceive it that way.

The recommendation to avoid stress is also not a valid way to reduce stress if one wants to live a full life. Only by adjusting our mental perspective about the situation can we actually avoid the stress in a healthy manner.

The recommendation to monitor stress may have back-fired as monitoring without an ability to change the situation (or perception of the situation) has the potential to increase stress. The awareness of high levels of stress and the potential negative health effects of that stress without a release valve would increase stress. That creates stress about being stressed.

Some individuals give up activities they enjoy because of time stress. Our pleasurable pursuits contribute to our health and resilience by providing a stress relief valve that helps us maintain stasis.

The recommendations provided in the 1970's were about as helpful to the typical individual as telling a pessimist to "think positively." Pessimism is a habit, not an inborn personality trait, but it is an insidious habit that is difficult to break without some knowledge and skills. With the knowledge and skills, anyone determined to become more optimistic is able to do so. Without the knowledge and skills, it seems impossible.

Additional research has been done and some of the recommendations being made today are more helpful. Some help reduce stress for brief periods and one (meditation) is effective both immediately and long-term.

But today's advice has still fallen far short of best practices. For the most part, it addresses symptoms rather than the root cause of stress.

The concept of positive thinking has become a common refrain. Sadly, the 'how' is usually absent when the advice is given. Imagine giving someone who was raised by wolves a book and telling him to read it—without teaching him to read. Telling a pessimist to think positively is not much different. Teach the individual how—in either situation—and the goal becomes attainable.

Although some individuals evolve optimistically, or learn it from a positively focused parent or grandparent, once pessimistic habits are developed, the opportunity to be optimistic without conscious knowledge is greatly diminished. Even today, many simply refer to the benefits of positivity and optimism and encourage people to think positively, but fail to provide knowledge and skills to help the person achieve the goal.

This often increases the level of stress because the person is now aware that being pessimistic is not in their best interest, but they do not have the skills and knowledge to change the pessimism it took a lifetime to develop. No mention was made, at that time, of the human ability to adjust ones mindset to reduce stress—the easiest response—also often the only one an individual has any control over[67].

The absence of the answer to the how question is what motivated me to create Happiness 1st Institute—because life is better when you are happy first. The techniques being taught—from gratitude, affirmations, meditation, exercise, helping others, being in nature, and others—all have some benefit. Real change, changes in the default responses, requires a deeper level of knowledge—a level where the student understands why these things work. The chapter on filtered consciousness explains the impact. The processes section provides the how. Together, the knowledge and skills provided are sufficient for individuals to significantly reduce their stress. First, we provide information about cutting edge science that demonstrates that each of us has guidance that leads us away from harm and toward self-actualization.

The first question most people ask when they hear we have guidance is why the world is not thriving if we have this guidance. The answer is that society habitually teaches us to misinterpret the guidance we receive and put other information ahead of our guidance. What the guidance means, the correct way to interpret it, and the healthiest way to respond to its messages is our next topic.

This path is simple enough to teach to children. In fact, they are born understanding the path and parents, teachers, church leaders, and society—who are well meaning, but ill-informed—teach them to ignore the simple path.

EGS refers to our **Emotional Guidance System**[68]. EGSc refers to the *Emotional Guidance Scale*. A sample scale is included in this chapter. It is helpful to keep a copy of the scale handy. The desire to feel happy or joyful is strong, but when we are at the lower end of the scale then attempting to reach those emotions will typically result in failure—if we attempt to get there in one step. The most successful method is to simply reach for a better feeling thought, which will give you a sense of relief from the tension (stress) you are feeling.

The scale is very beneficial because it is easiest to move up one emotional level at a time—and certainly not more than one zone at a time. That does not mean we have to remain in a lower emotional state for a long time. Generally, an individual who has some experience shifting perspectives to feel better can move up fairly rapidly—one step at a time. The definition of rapidly varies depending on the circumstances and level of experience. It can mean as little as less than a minute to a day or two or three.

That may not sound fast but compared to the typical situation, where movement only occurs when circumstances change and some people remain in lower emotional states for years, even a week is fast. Early in my own journey, I went from feeling so devastated by the end of a relationship that I could not talk about it without choking sobs to feeling ready to move on with my life in one weekend. A few years later, at the end of another relationship, I did not suffer the feelings of emotional devastation. The difference was that by then I knew there was a silver lining, so within minutes I was reaching for the better-feeling thoughts that come with knowing there was an upside.

After that, my ability to love fully and fearlessly was firmly entrenched. When you do not fear a bad ending, you can savor the relationship without doubt.

New scientific research shows us that our emotions are output from a hitherto unrecognized sense.[69] In fact, the emotional sense is present even in simple organisms. It appears that the function of basic "negative" emotions is to provide information necessary to the safety and well-being of the body. The function of positive emotions is to guide us toward self-development and well-being.[70]

The difference between simple organisms and most humans is that simple organisms always respond to their emotional sensory output. Simple organisms do not tolerate something that feels less than optimal any longer than necessary. Humans, on the other hand, often ignore or suppress their emotions and suffer the negative consequences of doing so by living lives that are less robust than they could be.[71]

Chapter 11: Emotional Guidance Sensory Feedback System (EGS)

Emotional Guidance Scale (EGSc)

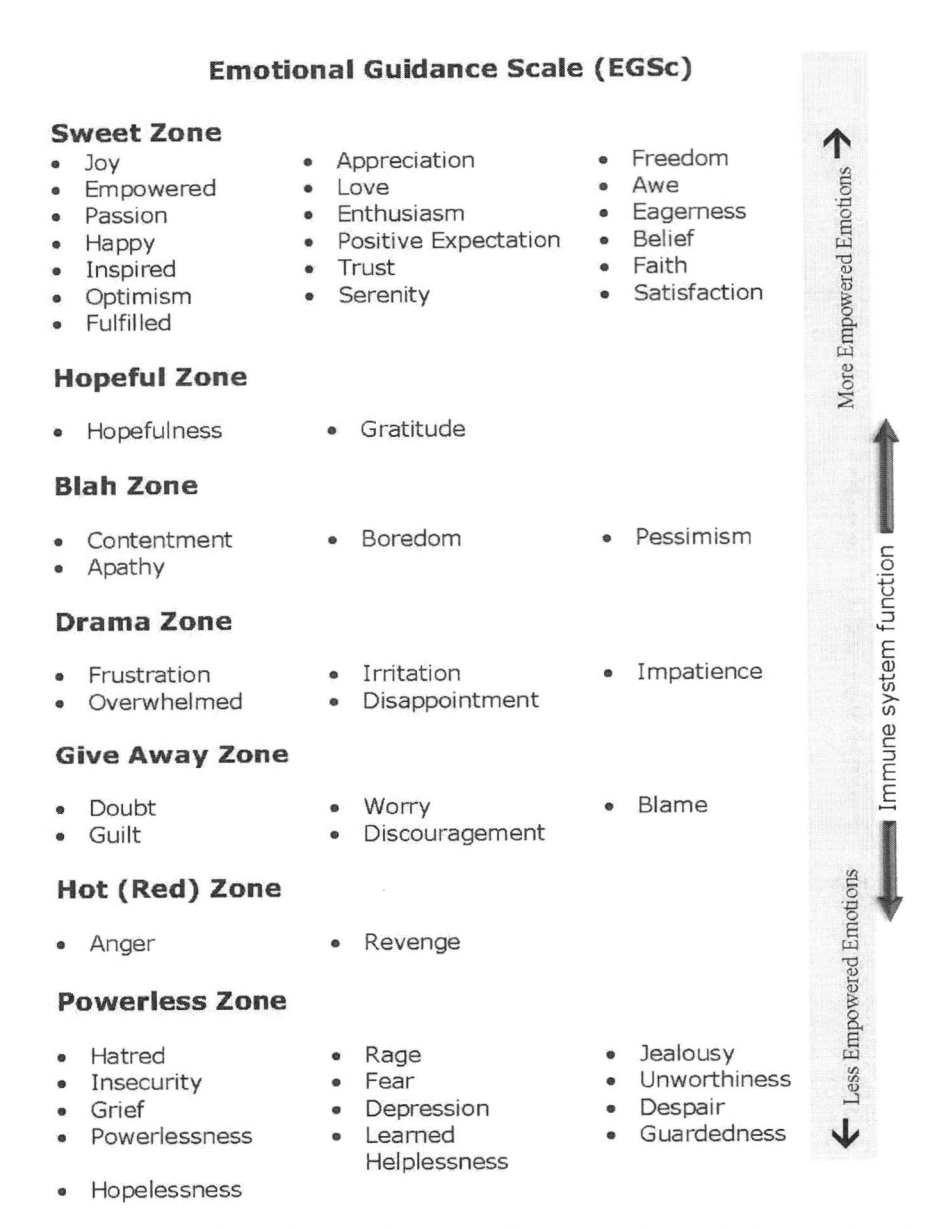

Sweet Zone
- Joy
- Empowered
- Passion
- Happy
- Inspired
- Optimism
- Fulfilled
- Appreciation
- Love
- Enthusiasm
- Positive Expectation
- Trust
- Serenity
- Freedom
- Awe
- Eagerness
- Belief
- Faith
- Satisfaction

Hopeful Zone
- Hopefulness
- Gratitude

Blah Zone
- Contentment
- Apathy
- Boredom
- Pessimism

Drama Zone
- Frustration
- Overwhelmed
- Irritation
- Disappointment
- Impatience

Give Away Zone
- Doubt
- Guilt
- Worry
- Discouragement
- Blame

Hot (Red) Zone
- Anger
- Revenge

Powerless Zone
- Hatred
- Insecurity
- Grief
- Powerlessness
- Hopelessness
- Rage
- Fear
- Depression
- Learned Helplessness
- Jealousy
- Unworthiness
- Despair
- Guardedness

↑ More Empowered Emotions

↕ Immune system function

↓ Less Empowered Emotions

People gain no benefit from ignoring the output from their emotional system. Emotions provide information that will improve people's lives if they act upon it appropriately. Ignoring negative emotional output is no different from ignoring pain from one's sense of touch. Emotional pain should be responded to in much the same way physical pain is managed. When emotional pain is ignored or suppressed, it can be as harmful to our well-being as leaving a burning hand on a hot stove.

Learning to follow the guidance from our EGS may conflict with instructions received throughout life For example, the opinions, expectations, and desires of others. In a world that does not currently understand the EGS, it is common for others to want you to behave in ways that make them happy. On the surface, it sounds very selfish to follow one's own guidance over what others may desire from you. By setting goals that include being loving, respectful to others, or to have good relationships, the EGS will provide guidance that considers these goals. Emotional guidance opens the door to a path to resilience that is simple and sure.

Our emotions are output from a sensory system. By heeding the guidance emotions provide, one increases their level of resilience.[72] Emotions provide information about whether we are moving toward or away from our best interests. While people have labeled emotions that feel bad as "negative" and those that feel good as "positive," all emotions are good because they are providing guidance, whether the receiver understands the message or the appropriate response to the message, or not. Emotions that do not feel good indicate action should be taken to feel better; action can be actual physical action or may consist of changing the perception that is leading to the emotion that does not feel good.

The research is clear that we have more to give to others when we are happy. Our EGS guides us to happier states. The increased resilience we gain from following our guidance can greatly benefit our families, employers, and communities.

In Peil's groundbreaking paper, "Emotion: A Self-regulatory Sense," she clearly demonstrates the importance of heeding the messages from the emotional sensory system. The paper also points to the true nature of humans and of the simplicity of following the Emotional Guidance System. Humans are good at the core of who they really are. However, it is only when they follow their emotional guidance that this is demonstrated consistently. When they do not follow their emotional guidance, behaviors that society does not favor can be the result.

> Emotions are information designed to guide us.

Peil's theory expands the responses to negative emotion from Fight or Flight to include Right Responses. Right Responses (RRs) should be the first response to most of the negative emotion experienced in modern life. There are different types of Right Responses, one is:

> *"...to affect the internal environment in the personal mindscape, in conscious knowledge acquisition, in an act of deliberate learning and personal mental tactic to invoke optimal belief structures to reappraise."*[73]

In other words, reach for a different perspective about the situation, one that feels better, and adopt that perspective because it serves your highest good to do so. Peil elaborates and clarifies the difference between a RR and suppressing emotions,

> *"There is a vast difference between a RR and suppressive emotion regulation, as the corrective action itself is informed*

by the specific emotional message, is consciously undertaken and it self-preserves through open, approach behavior, adaptive development and social cooperation. In short, the RR is a self-developmental response more indicative of the neurally well-endowed, culturally creative human being."

The knowledge and skills necessary to become adept at utilizing Right Responses are easily learned. The skills increase the level of positive emotions experienced by individuals—daily and over time—thus reducing stress and increasing their level of resilience.[74]

Teaching someone, even a child, to follow her own emotional guidance is simple. As Maia demonstrated to Marcello, the method resembles a simple children's game. There are myriad variations in the situations it can improve. It takes practice to respond consciously using RRs in the midst of a situation. However, in time it can become the default response.

If you have ever had a "Hell Yes" experience, it was your guidance shouting encouragement. I have had several. Yes, your guidance could have told you that someone you are now divorced from was a "Hell Yes" to marry. I know that from our perspective that seems wrong but sometimes the shortest path to where you really want to go involves what appears to be a wrong turn. The key is to take the good, the silver lining, and leave the unpleasant parts out. If you felt the "Hell Yes," it was on your best path to what you wanted.

Sometimes you can see what that was—or at least make a guess that feels right (which to me is the same thing). Sometimes you will never know. I was on an Alaskan cruise a few years ago. After the cruise, I planned to spend a few extra days in Seattle. Mid-way through the cruise I began having a strong urge to go home as soon as the cruise was over. I changed my flight and went home early. I have never learned why my guidance encouraged the change of plans, but I trust that it was the right path at that time.

Other times, I have known why. For instance, a few years later my fiancée and I were booked for a cruise and we both began feeling we should not take the trip. We cancelled and my Fiancée's father died when we would have been on the trip. I enjoy several vacations each year and that is the only one I have ever cancelled after it was booked.

Truly, the best way to understand how strong one's faith can be is to consider how strong our belief is when another sense has convinced us of its truth. If we see something, we tend to believe it. If we hear something, we tend to believe we heard it. If we touch something, we tend to believe what our sense of touch tells us about it. If we smell something, we believe it smells the way our nose interprets it.

Emotions are sensory feedback from our oldest sense. The only reason we do not trust them as much as our eyes, ears, nose and touch is that we have been trained not to trust them. Yet, when interpreted accurately, emotional feedback is the most accurate sense.

The myth that negative emotion means something outside ourselves is bad is commonly believed. It is responsible for significant amounts of unnecessary stress every day. Negative emotion means we are looking at something from a perspective that is less than ideal, or that we should focus elsewhere.

Let's look at a difficult situation for an example of alternative ways to perceive an event. Imagine a law enforcement officer working a murder investigation. If the job required the officer to focus on the loss felt by loved ones, the experiences the victim will miss in the future, and other aspects that feel awful, the negative emotion would quickly prostrate the officer. I am not saying officers do not think about these things, I am saying their job does not require them to focus on these aspects.

The job requires a problem-solving attitude. When gruesome details are the focus, the perspective is in relationship to answering the question, "What will this tell me that will help solve this case?" The focus on future action feels better in comparison to focusing on an unchangeable past event. The focus on solving the mystery feels better than a focus on a life ended too soon. The focus on providing answers to the family feels better than thinking about all the times the family will miss their loved one in the future.

The negative emotion is not saying the situation is bad. Nor is it saying it is good. The negative emotion is communicating that there is a way to perceive the situation that is more in alignment with our personal goals. A law enforcement officer choosing to focus on the aspects of a case that feel the worse will not be able to achieve the goal of solving the case. Her cognitive function will be impaired. Her immune system will be depressed. Choosing the worse feeling perception will not advance the goal of solving the case. A mental stance of hopefulness that the case will be solved supports the cognitive function required to accomplish the task—and is accompanies by better feeling emotional responses.

We have the ability to choose the way we perceive any event. Our EGS guides us to the one that gives us the best chance of achieving our goal.

With practice we can learn to trust our emotional guidance as much as, or more than, our other senses. Once that level of trust develops, life improves immeasurably. This is because our emotions take into consideration information available on the quantum level that our other senses cannot consider.

For example, our EGS considers others' intentions. While our eyes might catch a glimmer of intent through body language, accurately interpreting body language is a science that few have mastered. Likewise, our ears might sense something in the tone of voice, but unless we are experts, we may not trust our interpretation. If we were experts at determining truth from lies in the spoken word, we would not need a machine to detect lies. Interpreting and trusting our EGS is far easier than becoming an expert in body language and the nuances contained in various tones of voice.

Chapter 11: Emotional Guidance Sensory Feedback System (EGS)

Without an understanding of one's guidance, it would be extremely hard to have enough faith in things that do not make sense and that one cannot see clearly from lower emotional levels. With an understanding of one's guidance, faith can be strong and sure, unshakable, and certainly not in need of validation by someone else.

For example, this morning a young couple had an interaction during which it sounded as if the Fern was upset at Bob when he asked if she would join him in an activity they both enjoy. Bob interpreted it as if Fern was upset with him for asking and his feelings were somewhat hurt, as he had no idea why she was being prickly. Fern declined his invitation because she had responsibilities to tend take care of. She was not upset with Bob, but with the fact that her duties made it necessary to forgo the desired activity with him. Her reason was almost polar opposite to the reason he perceived (upset with him) whereas she was upset not to be able to join him.

Utilizing my guidance to interpret what was really going on, I was able to know, with certainty, that there had been a miscommunication. I let them know how it was misinterpreted and clarified the intent of the female. I then asked each of them to correct me if I was in any way wrong. "Nope, you nailed it," was the reply.

How many times a day do misunderstandings like this interfere with the smooth functioning of an office environment? How much more productive would it be if the employees could use their guidance to check on the others' intent. Even better, if the employees understood that even if someone intended to be rude, their behavior has far more to do with their own emotional state than it does with anyone they are interacting with. The employees would be empowered not to take it personally. After all, it is not personal. If the co-worker were happy, he would not be rude.

The lack of knowledge of the EGS and thus society's failure to use it leads to many problems, from simple misunderstandings to wars between nations. In more traditional relationships and lifestyles, the desire to have ones choices validated by others is evidenced by disagreements that often become divisive.

Regardless of the choices a person makes, there are usually people who disagree with the choice. We are surrounded by examples, including single Mom, working Mom, stay-at-home Dad, public school, private school, structured activities or free play, make your bed every day, don't make your bed every day, mow your grass to 2" or mow it to 4", eat meat, don't eat meat, and more. Having choices is good, but expecting everyone else to make the same choice we make creates conflict.

At the root of it all is a defensiveness born of insecurity. Because they do not use their guidance, they feel an unsatisfied desire to have their decisions validated. The desire for validation is natural. We are born with guidance that provides validation. When we have a "Hell Yes" experience, we are receiving validation from our EGS loud and clear. When we do not receive the validation, we can become quite upset—because we inherently feel that our choices should be validated. We have been looking in the wrong place for validation. Our guidance is where that need should be satisfied. Our guidance is validating our choices when they are correct for us and letting us know when they differ from our best path. But if we do not recognize the guidance for what it is, we do not gain the satisfaction of feeling validated.

This discord is seen in every area of life. It is common in religion, politics, and even music. A great deal of time, effort, and stress results from attempting to demand conformity.

Actions that someone with a belief that the world is a good place would interpret one way, someone who believes they live in an evil world will interpret extremely differently.

This points to another reason there are so many conflicts, and why it could be so hard to convince people of something that others could see clearly. People are taught that their minds are rational. They are encouraged to trust their mind over their emotions. The emotional guidance is not filtered by ones beliefs. It is often difficult to understand its messages once one has been trained to believe the rational mind is the better source of decision-making. But, it is not hard to straighten out with a little bit of effort and practice using ones emotional guidance.

Using a dual system for decision-making, by using both the rational brain and emotional guidance for the same decisions and giving their EGS more weight in areas that do not seem important develops confidence. By beginning in this way, it soon becomes clear that the guidance from the EGS leads to better outcomes. Many students quickly begin giving greater weight to the EGS.

What are some of the ways we are taught to misinterpret our guidance? From young ages, many of us are taught to ignore or suppress our guidance. When we were two and our brother took our toy away, Mom did not show us how to feel better using our guidance. She distracted us by giving us another toy. Or she told us, "Don't cry. You're alright." While those may not be considered bad ways to parent, and they are certainly superior to the angry parent who smacks her child for crying, they ignore the guidance the child was born with. The first technique teaches the child the parent will make him feel better when he is upset. The lesson the child learns is: *"Finding a way to feel better is not your job. Mom will do it for you."* In the second example, the message is: *"Expressing your emotions is not good behavior. Suppress them."* Emotions become bothersome things that we have to deal with instead of the valuable tool they are.

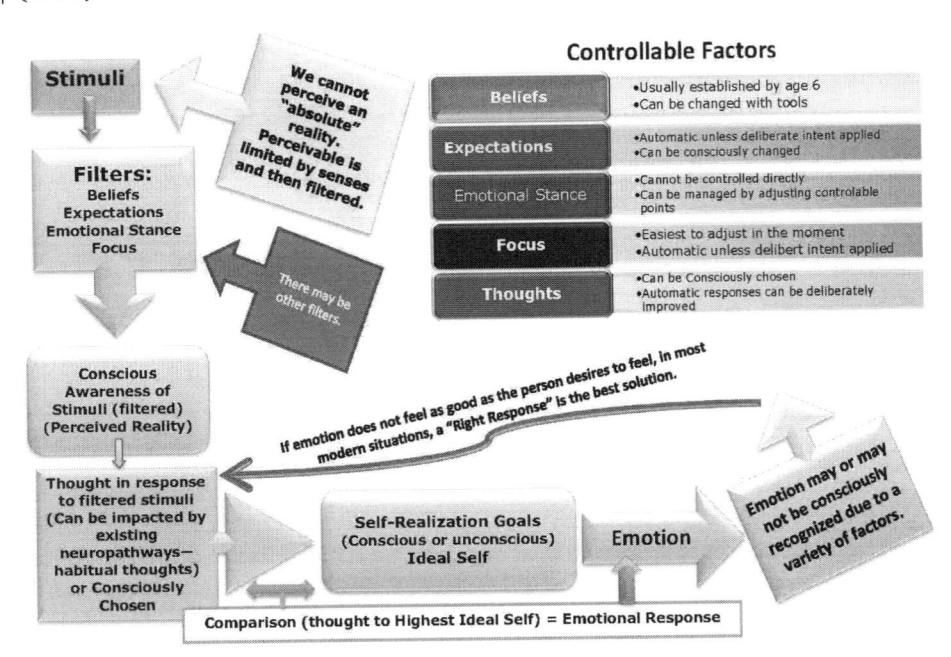

Chapter 11: Emotional Guidance Sensory Feedback System (EGS)

Stimuli

We cannot perceive an "absolute" reality. Perceivable is limited by senses and then filtered.

Filters:
Beliefs
Expectations
Emotional Stance
Focus

There may be other filters.

Conscious Awareness of Stimuli (filtered) (Perceived Reality)

Thought in response to filtered stimuli (Can be impacted by existing neuropathways—habitual thoughts) or Consciously Chosen

If emotion does not feel as good as the person desires to feel, in most modern situations, a "Right Response" is the best solution.

Controllable Factors

Beliefs	• Usually established by age 6 • Can be changed with tools
Expectations	• Automatic unless deliberate intent applied • Can be consciously changed
Emotional Stance	• Cannot be controlled directly • Can be managed by adjusting controllable points
Focus	• Easiest to adjust in the moment • Automatic unless delibert intent applied
Thoughts	• Can be Consciously chosen • Automatic responses can be deliberately improved

Self-Realization Goals (Conscious or unconscious) Ideal Self

Emotion — Emotion may or may not be consciously recognized due to a variety of factors.

Comparison (thought to Highest Ideal Self) = Emotional Response

---

Emotions are our friend. We should understand them as messages letting us know if we are moving in the direction we want to go. We should understand our power to change our emotional stance by changing our perception of any situation. When I say "any situation," many people want to argue that some situations are just so awful that there is no way to find a better feeling perception. As long as someone has that belief, they won't find it. In his book *Infinite Love and Gratitude*, Dr. Darrell Weismann writes about how he found a better perspective about his daughter's death and how doing so helped the wound heal.

No one would wish for that situation but many live through it. A book I found especially helpful after my first miscarriage was, *Ho for California!: Pioneer Women and Their Quilts* by Jean Ray Laury and the California Heritage Quilt Project. The book chronicles quilts that came to California, by wagon train, around the horn and, if memory serves, by train. The great value I found in it was the strength of the women, some of whom birthed a dozen children and lost over half of them before they reached adulthood. That these women could suffer losses like that and still function, much less leave a lasting legacy in the form of a quilt, helped me see the potential for resilience within each of us.

Once something happens that must be lived through, there is a choice. Live through it and celebrate your life, perhaps giving greater meaning to your child's life, or choose a path of suffering. Another example of a parent who brought meaning to her daughter's death is the founder of MADD, Cindy Lightner. Although I am sure no parent would ever choose to sacrifice their child, the fact that MADD has been instrumental in decreasing DUI fatalities by about 50%, saving 12,000 lives each year must bring some solace and meaning to her loss.

There is a way for anyone, in any circumstances, to move forward. If you are currently suffering, I do not know your path forward—but your EGS does know. It is with you 24/7 providing feedback in response to your every thought. Find the one that feels better. Soak it in until you feel stable in holding that thought and then reach for one that feels even better.

I've met many people in my life who are actually afraid of what they will find if they explore too much of their inner world. Somewhere along the way they have been convinced the possibility they are evil could be hiding inside them. Peil's paper suggests the true nature of humans: they are good at the core of who they really are. Seligman echoes this argument in *Flourish* and Dacher Keltner reinforces it in *Born to be Good*.

However, only when emotional guidance is followed consistently is our true nature demonstrated.[75] Prolonged negative emotions that result when the emotional guidance system is ignored can lead to undesirable behaviors. We feel emotions in response to thoughts. Even when our body communicates, for example, the physical hair standing up on the back of the neck in response to danger, it is not until we consciously recognize that we feel the hair standing up, a thought about the physical manifestation that fear is felt.

> "I do not think stress is a legitimate topic of conversation, in public anyway. No one ever wants to hear how stressed anyone else is, because most of the time everyone is stressed out. Going on and on in detail about how stressed I am isn't conversation. It'll never lead anywhere."
> Mindy Kaling
>
> This quote reflects how many people feel about stress. But I think it goes deeper—there is an inner urge to help the stressed person but they're so stressed themselves they feel they don't have time to help—and they don't really know how to help. When society understands that help means helping the individuals find a better-feeling thought and they know the EGSc, they know the path to a better thought, helping will be easy. I do it all the time and it brings me great joy to uplift others as I move through my days.
> The not knowing how to help is what brings the discomfort. We can change that.

Chapter 11: Emotional Guidance Sensory Feedback System (EGS)

I see a distinct difference between the fear that makes the hair on the back of your neck stand up and the fear you feel when someone tells you a story about something awful happening to someone you have never met. Fight or flight is an appropriate response when the hair on the back of your neck is standing up. A Right Response is a more appropriate response to the second type of stress. This distinction is important in a world with 24/7 news scouring the planet and looking for every awful thing that has happened around the world.

Far more goes right in the world, every day, than goes wrong. If we put the worlds' troubles in the perspective of our body with the bad things in proportion to the good, the world has a hang nail. I am not saying awful things aren't happening. I am saying that filing your head with them as you begin your evening and/or as you head to bed is not healthy for you. It does not solve the problem. In almost every situation there is nothing you can do. But what do most people do? They feel fear. Look at where fear is on the EGS. The fear is increased when loved ones, especially teenagers and young adults are out or away at college.

The 24/7 negative news has primed most of us to be afraid of this beautiful world we live in. Many will argue that they have to be realistic. Viewing a minute percentage of the things happening on the planet is not at all realistic—it is a view with a major negative bias. If the 24/7 news channels reported good news and bad news in proportion to their occurrence, the bad news would last less than a minute each day.

If you are feeling you live in a bad world, I encourage you to shift your focus to one that is more realistic. Start with the big picture and get as specific as you can while still feeling good. The sun came up today. Even if it was on the other side of clouds, the sun rose today. The atmosphere is filled with air I can breathe. Wow! Two huge, necessary hurdles done! Are the birds singing? Are the plants growing? Is the sun feeding the plants? Are the clouds watering the plants? Did people fall in love today? Did people hold hands today? Were any babies born today? I have two eyes that see, two ears that hear, one nose, two arms, two legs complete with feet. I have family I love, who love me. I have friends I love, who love me. I have a bed and a kitchen and windows. I have guidance that responds to every thought I think. I could go on like this for an entire book so I'll stop now. You get the idea. The amount of wonderful going on, every day, is enormous. So be realistic, think positive.

One more point about the news. Have you considered what the job of the news stations is? Follow the money. They are paid for ratings. Researchers figured out a long time ago that if you make people fearful they watch the news more often. How do you get ratings higher? More viewers equals higher ratings!

Don't take my word for it. Use your own guidance to make your decision.

Emotions are responses to thoughts.[76] Each thought elicits an emotional response. [77,78 & 79]Emotional guidance is unique to the individual thinking the thought. Unique goals, beliefs, expectations, emotional stances and focuses cause differences in the emotional responses individuals receive. When we move away from our goals, our emotions feel worse. By deliberately choosing a different perspective, our thoughts change and better-feeling emotions can be deliberately cultivated.[80] Thoughts actually create meaning for events in life. [81] For example, if someone cancels an appointment the individual who is told the meeting will not occur is free to assign meaning to the event. Even when a reason is given, the reason may or may not be accepted by the receiver. If the reason is not accepted, the individual will create a reason to explain the event to himself. That explanation may be one that feels good or one that feels bad. Whichever is chosen, the event will be experienced (felt emotionally) by the individual as if the assigned reason is true.

It is really as simple as understanding that better feeling thoughts are guiding us toward our desires and thoughts that feel worse are advising us that we are moving away from our desires. Some clarity regarding desires is required. There is a difference between short term and long term desires. Although all desires contain the characteristic that we believe we will feel better in the attaining of them, some desires relate to immediate gratification; a response to current conditions without consideration for the long term. Desires for some foods, drugs, alcohol, and other addictions are fueled by these types of desires. Short-term desires are often accompanied by conflicting emotions caused by conflicts with longer term desires. For example, a desire to feel better right now may be satisfied by enjoyment of a piece of chocolate cake but the desire to maintain a comfortable weight in the long term may be in direct conflict with that desire.

There is an inherent desire to feel better. Many 'desires' are not beneficial in the long term. Without knowledge of techniques to change thoughts, endless loops can result—sugary foods, alcohol, drugs, shopping and more can temporarily improve mood, but do not build long-term resilience. To build long-term resilience one must reach for better feeling thoughts. The more attention that is given to long term goals, the more they will be considered in the emotional response you receive when a short-term goal seems to conflict with the long-term goals.

For example, in an upsetting situation it is not uncommon for individuals to reach for alcohol to provide relief from their negative emotions. Unfortunately, alcohol provides only a temporary dulling of the pain (or lessening of the focus on the painful thoughts) and can lead to even greater problems.

A more permanent method of approaching an upsetting situation is to reframe ones perception of the event in a way that feels better.[82] With practice, finding better feeling thoughts becomes easier in many adverse situations.

Chapter 11: Emotional Guidance Sensory Feedback System (EGS)

> *"No beating yourself up. That's not allowed. Be patient with yourself. It took you years to form the bad habits of thought that you no longer want. It will take a little time to form new and better ones. I promise you this: Even a slight move in this direction will bring you some peace. The more effort you apply to it, the faster you'll find your bliss, but you'll experience rewards immediately."*
> — Holly Mosier

It is possible to maintain a positive bias about life when circumstances are not ideal. This has been proven by many in very adverse circumstances. There are many accounts; one of the most dire is the story of Viktor Frankl, documented in his book, *Man's Search for Meaning*, about his experiences in a Nazi concentration camp. In the worst of circumstances he discovered the importance of finding meaning in all forms of existence, which made his current circumstances, even though unchanged and reprehensible, feel better and provided a reason to continue living. This is an example of a RR, where the individual found better-feeling thoughts. Although the thoughts he found were philosophical in nature, any thoughts that felt better and thus made the situation more tolerable would be considered RRs.

Science has tended to study various aspects of humanity in isolation (Psychology, biochemistry, medical, neurological, consciousness, behavioral, sociology, criminology, genetics, physics, etc.). These areas of science are often subdivided into specialties, such as addiction, immunology, cardiovascular disease, beliefs, epigenetics, and more.

It is all interrelated. Root cause solutions require an understanding of the larger picture.

Thoughts create the emotional feedback. The emotional stance affects body chemistry, bodily processes, behaviors/actions, and ultimate outcomes.

Circumstances do not create the emotion. There is evidence from individuals who live in far less advantageous circumstances who are happy with their lives and receive the benefits of positivity. Research into disparate outcomes in situations with homogenous incomes vs. situations with greater differences reflects that it is not actual circumstances, but perception thereof that matters.

Likewise, there are many stories of cancer survivors who claim that being diagnosed with cancer was the best thing that ever happened to them. The reasons vary, but most of the individuals learned to live more consciously instead of being content with an "auto-pilot" life[83], where they merely react to their circumstances without any knowledge that they can control how they respond to events. "With the cancer diagnosis, my priorities changed in an instant. The list of what was truly important got real short, real quick. Decision-making became easier. I became more motivated to do things I had been putting off. The old phrase about not sweating the small stuff became crystal clear."[84]

Human societies train people to "keep a stiff upper lip" and to "be strong" by which they mean endure negative emotions instead of finding better feeling thoughts.

A change of perception changes everything. Each mind interprets the world according to factors specific to the individual,[85] including beliefs, expectations, emotional stance, and focus. These factors create a filtering system in the brain that determines the sensory input that is communicated to the conscious mind. People project their thoughts onto what they see and experience in the world. When one changes her thoughts, her world changes. People give thoughts power when they accept them as true. Everyone has a choice. Right Responses involve deliberately changing beliefs, expectations, and focus.

In a recent study[86] of individuals experiencing divorce, self-compassion—which would translate into less negative self-talk—was cited as the factor that uniquely predicts good outcomes.

Several branches of science have been studying human thriving. The results, when compiled, point to the fact that people thrive when they feel emotionally good and suffer when they do not[87].

When individuals know they have this guidance, and have practiced using it, they also know that no matter how bad their current circumstances may seem, they can find ways to feel better. Hope, a belief that a positive or desired outcome is possible, is a key emotional state for resilience. Just knowing that guidance exists builds a firm foundation for hopefulness[88]. Without this knowledge, it is easier to feel hopeless, which can lead to inertia or giving up[89].

The following chart was developed to point out that individuals who developed certain behaviors were more resilient. In many ways, the statement that individuals who develop the more resilient behaviors feel less stress in the same circumstances.

Chapter 11: Emotional Guidance Sensory Feedback System (EGS)

Less Resilient	More Resilient
Disempowered perspective	→ Empowered perspective [90]
Sees problems as permanent	→ Expects to bounce back [91]
Victim thinking	→ Refuses victim mindset [92]
Blames	→ Accepts responsibility [93]
Feels fearful/helpless	→ Feels confidence/capable
Responds reactively	→ Consciously chooses perspective
Rigid thinking	→ Feels curiosity
Holds onto anger	→ Forgives easily
Resistance to new ideas	→ Welcomes new ideas & experiences [94]
Feels hopeless	→ Feels hopeful
Expects the worse	→ Faith
Tendency to attack oneself	→ Belief in Self & Ability to learn [95]
Holds onto guilt	→ Characterizes failure as learning [96]
Feelings of shame	→ Self-Acceptance and Approval [97]
Negative emotional bias	→ Positive emotional bias [98]
Long-term worry and anxiety	→ Trust
Being "right" is highest goal	→ Places higher goals above "being right" [99]
Feels life "just happens"	→ Feels Personal Control [100]
Sees obstacles as enemies	→ Obstacles are challenges [101] (opportunities)

I am often asked to explain the source of the guidance. Realistically—it does not matter. Our guidance guides us toward our individual goals and toward our highest good. Experimenting with your guidance makes it clear it guides us around obstacles and toward goals. Sometimes faith is required because the path the mind wants us to take seems more logical but when our guidance is followed we usually, eventually, learn why the straightest path is where our guidance feels best. Our guidance helps us be more of who we want to be.

Where it comes from is another matter. Quantum physics provided many of the answers. The research into biophotons and cellular communication using light are illuminating. There is much that is not known yet. I strongly encourage readers to experiment with their own EGS because in this experience is the only way to know for sure that the guidance is beneficial, accurate, and always present.

In Chapter 12 of *Perspectives on Coping and Resilience*, I detail my research into whether common religions including Buddhist, Christianity, Islam, Hindu, and Confucius support guidance. Another book is underway for the spiritual but not religious community. Since over than 90% of us have a worldview that is influenced by our religious and/or spiritual beliefs, it is important to understand if they support the science and if the science supports them.

As previously cited, positive emotions are immensely beneficial for us—increasing our resilience, reducing the risks from negative life events, decreasing the risk of all types of major illnesses and improving relationships. We have an EGS that helps us enjoy better-feeling emotions. It makes sense to understand and use the guidance available to us.

Chapter 11: Emotional Guidance Sensory Feedback System (EGS)

Chapter 12: Filtered Consciousness

Reality is merely an illusion, albeit a very persistent one.
Albert Einstein

Our consciousness does not perceive an actual reality[102]. The reality our minds perceive is filtered[103]. This chapter will explain the main filters that impact our perception of reality.

When I have written about a topic in a way that feels just right, it is better to use it than attempt to reinvent the wheel. I begin this chapter by sharing part of a speech I wrote for a day-long peace rally. It will help if you imagine yourself in a large, crowded auditorium as you read the next few pages.

> *The first thing I will speak of is the function of our minds.*
>
> *We are taught to believe our minds. Let me ask you some questions.*
>
> *Until this moment, when I mention it, do you feel your clothing?*
>
> *Unless you are experiencing a binding or itchy clothes day, the answer was no.*
>
> *Yet, I do not see anyone who is naked in the audience.*
>
> *Do you think your skin was not feeling your clothing? Or do you think your brain said something like, "If I continually send reminders about what the skin is feeling, it will take up too much capacity. That capacity is needed for things that are currently being focused on?" Because our brains are expert resource managers—they filter the*

information our sense of touch receives about our clothing so the data was not transferred to our conscious mind.

Yes, or yes?

If any of you are holding hands with a loved one, how much are you noticing you are holding hands?

Isn't it when the hands move, when they caress, that you feel the touch?

Right now, turn to your neighbor. Touch one another's hands.

Do you not feel the sense of touch?

But, if you remain there, after a while, when you are comfortable, you will not feel it unless you focus on it.

Right, or right?

It's a cold day. On days like this, I love to put dinner in the crock-pot and let it cook all day. I sometimes work from home. When I do, I do not notice the wonderful aroma of my dinner cooking.

But, when I go outside to bring in the mail and return, the aroma is strong when I enter the house.

Yet, after I am back inside for a minute or so, I no longer smell them. Do you think my nose stops working?

Does your nose work the same way?

Sometimes that is a good thing, yes?

If I continually smelled the delicious aroma while I was trying to work, would it interfere with my productivity?

Maybe.

Probably.

Let me ask you another question. When I am working at home with a fine roast in the crockpot, what is my reality? In reality, does my home smell delicious? If a visitor walks in, will they not smell the aroma? Yet, in my personal reality, I do not smell it. Is my nose broken? Or, is there a filter between my conscious mind and the information my senses receive?

Whether I am not feeling my clothing, not smelling dinner, or not feeling the chair I am sitting on—reality has not changed. My senses are aware of them. My conscious perception of reality is being filtered. What causes my mind to filter these things? When dinner is in the crockpot and I have been in the house a while, can I inhale and smell the aroma if I think about it? Yes, I can. My nose still smells the aroma. It is just being filtered from what my conscious mind receives.

Our brain uses filters to decide which information is passed to our conscious mind. The four main filters are beliefs, expectations, emotional stance, and focus. These filters are important. They are tools we can use to make our lives better. They are very powerful.

In the chapter on Perception, you began understanding that the reality you experience is based on how you, personally, interpret reality[104]. Before you become consciously aware of anything in your life, the data you receive is filtered through these filters.

Before big data reaches your conscious mind it is mined for what is relevant—based on what the programming of your filters determines is important. Imagine a miner looking for sapphires but he has no idea what a diamond is. This miner is in your mind, scanning the big data (input from all your senses), finding sapphires, and sending the information to your conscious mind. When the miner sees a diamond, it goes in the irrelevant file—because the miner is not programmed to find diamonds.

Your beliefs are established by around age 6 and in the typical human, do not change much from the ones established at a young age[105]. Some adjustments might be made, but most are the result of experiences lived—which are interpreted after the input is filtered. We perceive reality in a way that supports our established beliefs.

Your filters are of enormous value to you. Millions of bits of information are received by your senses every second. You do not have the capability to pay attention to all the input so the information is filtered. The programming regarding what information is passed to your conscious mind is, in most individuals, an unconscious action that is programmed at a young age. However, at any time, we can choose to reprogram our filters in ways that serve us better.

For example, someone who has decided they are unlovable will attribute ulterior motives to the actions of others. The person cannot perceive love even when it is given freely, because it contradicts their belief that they are unlovable. Unless and until this individual changes the belief, he will not experience being loved. This will be true even with his wife and children. If he is successful, he may interpret the wife as being with him for financial reasons. He might have accepted this arrangement because he wanted to have companionship, children, sex, or give a public perception of normalcy. (This may have absolutely nothing to do with why she married him.) His wife may love him dearly but he will interpret her actions as if they are due to another motivation. His children will receive the same treatment. He might, seemingly out of the blue, complain that all the child wants him for is his financial support—with no basis in reality. In fact, even counter information does not override the strong belief that he is not lovable.

Someone who believes they are unlovable will never be able to feel loved unless and until they change their belief about being lovable. If this man were to shift his belief until he truly believed he was lovable, he would then interpret the actions of his wife and children through that filter and see them in an entirely different light.

Let's take this into the workplace and use an employee who believes she is not appreciated. It won't matter if you give her more appreciation than any two other employees combined, she will not feel appreciated. As long as she has a filter programmed with the belief "I am not appreciated" she will attribute the employer's appreciation to another motivation.

Likewise, if someone believes they are the best, no matter how much information (big data) exists indicating otherwise, the person will interpret reality as if he is the best. If someone whose performance is actually better is promoted ahead of him, he will not attribute it to the superior performance. In fact, he will not be able to perceive the others' performance as superior—often giving himself excuses for why his did not match the others' combined with a strong belief that if the playing field were equal, he would be better. For example, in sales, he might use the excuse that his territory did not have as much potential opportunity as the one who had the better performance in sales numbers. He will not attribute the others' promotion to higher skills because that would conflict with his belief that he is the best.

The same thing happens with appearance. If a beautiful woman does not believe she is beautiful, it will not matter how many times she is told she is beautiful. Each time, she will make up a reason (other than her beauty) that the person said she was beautiful. She will not experience the compliments emotionally the same way she would if she believed she was beautiful.

If she someday changes her perception of self and begins believing she is beautiful, the first time someone tells her she is beautiful after she believes it, she will experience the moment as if it is the first time she has ever heard that from another. In many ways, it is the first time she has heard it clearly. The other times were accompanied by negation from the voice in her head. "He's just saying that because he wants something" or "He's just saying that to make me feel good." The actual experience of being told she is beautiful and believing the words is a very different experience.

If you have ever wondered how or why highly successful people (think Hollywood as an example) are not happy, sometimes ruining their careers and even their lives, with drugs and alcohol, the root problem may be that they have underlying beliefs that are hindering the ability to enjoy their success.

There is a difference between striving to improve oneself because of a desire to be the best one can be and striving to improve because of a belief that one is not good enough. Michael Jordan reminds me of the individual who strives to improve himself because he has a desire to be his personal best. There is nothing wrong with striving to be our personal best. In fact, when we do that with a belief that we can achieve our goals, it is healthy and fulfilling, but if the striving is done from a position of lack, of not being good enough, the individual will never feel that he's reached the goal—no matter how good he becomes.

You know the saying "Statistics can be used to prove anything." Well, the same is true of the filters in our minds. They will prove to us whatever we believe.

Let's return to the speech:

> *Of the four main filters, focus is the easiest to adjust in any given moment. Adjusting your focus can change your emotional stance and, continually and deliberately adjusting your focus over time, changes your chronic emotional stance.*
>
> *Your brain does not care if the filters serve you or not. In fact, I believe that we are expected to understand how to set our filters to maximize our life experience, to help us attain our highest good. The filters are designed as if we understand how they work. The filters literally hide information that is inconsistent with how they are set—whether it is in our best interest or not. They are not malicious, vindictive, or determining our deservability or worthiness. Our belief about our worthiness creates a filter, which then determines how the filters process information. The judgment of anyone outside yourself about your worth does not change your filters. If you allow another's judgments to affect your beliefs about yourself, your filters adjust. The filters carry out their programming.*
>
> *I do not believe our minds would deliberately harm us yet they do when the filters are set to unhealthy or unproductive settings. I choose to believe that we were meant to understand how to set our filters to serve our highest good.*
>
> *When I mention beliefs, many people think I am speaking of their religious beliefs. While religious beliefs are beliefs, I am speaking of more than religious beliefs. I have*

no intention or desire to change any beliefs that are serving you.

I will not tell you what to think. Nor will I tell you what to believe. Your guidance will do that. My guidance is for my goals. Your goals and my goals are not going to be the same. Most of this room has no desire to stand up here on the stage. It is one of my biggest desires because it fulfills another, stronger desire—that of being able to help as many people as I can to thrive more in every area of their lives.

My guidance leads me to my goals. Yours leads you to yours.

If you have not consciously set goals, your guidance is muted. There are many factors that mute the guidance, but consciously setting goals increases the volume enough for some people that they begin thriving. That is why goal setting has remained an important business tool for decades. It works because it makes our guidance about the goals louder. By louder, I do not mean you will hear voices in your mind. I mean your thoughts will consider the goal. Your choices will consider the goal. The very thoughts you think are affected by goal setting. There are other ways to increase the volume even more than goal setting.

What is a belief?

A belief is just a thought you have thought repeatedly until a filter is established making it part of your reality. Just as I cannot smell the pot roast when I am in the house, belief filters filter out information that contradicts the belief from our reality.

That is why you can see something so clearly and someone else, with different beliefs, cannot see it no matter how clear your arguments may be.

You could have a burning question, maybe a solution to a health or employment crisis and have the answer on a piece of paper in your hand, but if you believe an answer does not exist, your brain will not make the connection between the solution in your hand and what you are seeking.

Yet, shift that belief to one that believes it is possible to find a solution, and you will see the solution.

Think about that. Think about looking for a job in an economy you believe makes it impossible to find a job if you're over 50, under 30, or whatever other criteria you've used to decide you can't find a job. It is true, for you. You can't find a job. But it is not the economy. There are those who thrive and those who suffer in every type of economy.

The reason some thrive is they believe they can.

The reason some suffer is they believe they cannot thrive.

The reasons they hold those beliefs do not matter The truth or falsity of the beliefs does not matter. Only the belief matters to the filtering system. The filters are adjusted to support our beliefs. The filters do not decide what is best for you, they just follow instructions.

If you believe something is true for yourself and not for others, that thing is a filter you established. You may not have done it deliberately, but you did do it. This is actually good news. We can adjust and control our filters. Just like driving a vehicle, when we know how to do it, we can keep it on the road we want to take.

Most of our beliefs are established by age 6. Most of us do not understand the filters, so we never consciously adjust them. We just suffer from poorly programmed filters. Because our brain's job is to prove our beliefs to us, the longer we live the more sure we are we are right. Our filters ensure we repeatedly interpret reality in a way that is consistent with our beliefs about reality.

Yet, if the belief is not true for everyone, it is merely that—a belief.

I want you to think to yourself—do not say it aloud about—the amount of annual salary you believe you are worth. The number I want you to think is not what you are paid, it is what you believe you are worth.

Now, think for a moment, to yourself, about why you make what you make. Pay attention to the first thought you have about why this number is more or less than what you think your work is worth.

Did you think you make your current salary because you are too much something or too little something?

Now, let me ask you some questions.

Do all people who make more than you have more education than you?

Are all people who make more than you smarter than you are?

Are all of the people who make more than you better than you do in terms of morals and ethics?

Are all the people who make more than you older than you are?

Are all the people who make more than you younger than you are?

Are all the people who make more than you born into wealthier families?

Are all the people who make more than you a different gender than you are?

Are all the people who make more than you a different race than you are?

Are all the people who make more than you prettier or more handsome?

Those are common excuses people use to explain why they can't make the income they believe they should.

Life is much better when we look for the reasons we can. We find what we look for.

A long time ago, I believed only people who knew secrets I had no idea how to learn made six figure incomes. Making that kind of money seemed mysterious to me. My mind did not dwell on the topic because it did not feel good to do so. But I remember thinking about it and feeling as if those who made that kind of income were somehow different than I was. It was not based on a label, to me it was more of a mysterious something I believed I lacked.

When I deliberately changed my belief and began believing I could make six figures my income increased 64% in a year and I was making over six figures. The only thing that changed was my belief. As a result of the belief change, I was able to recognize opportunities to achieve that goal. Before my belief changed, I would have self-selected myself out of the running, telling myself I was not ready or was not good enough. I would not have even tried. Once I believed I could do it, I tried and succeeded.

If the reason you believe you make less than you believe you are worth is one where you answered "no" to one of the above questions, you have identified a limiting belief. Sometimes individuals who learn they have a limiting belief, or about limiting beliefs, decide to go on a search and destroy mission to find and eliminate beliefs that are hindering their ability to thrive. Don't do that. It can take years and tends to have unsatisfactory results. Take the shortcut.

The shortcut is to decide which beliefs would serve you and develop those beliefs. Read about individuals you admire and wish to emulate. Pay attention to the way they think. Quotes can be very helpful. Using your EGS when you read a quote makes identifying ideas that make your heart sing and your pulse race easy. Your EGS will also identify beliefs that will not serve you by giving you negative emotion when you read it. When you find beliefs that you want the world to reflect back to you, take steps to believe them. Processes for this are in the Processes section of this book. Remember, a belief is simply a thought you have thought repeatedly until it becomes a habit of thought.

Your filters, if not set to maximize your thriving, will filter out opportunities that are available to you. If your beliefs do not make those opportunities part of your reality, you won't see them, you won't hear about them, and you won't benefit from them.

Right about now many of you are thinking "there's no way it was right in front of me I'd know about it and see it." But think about our focus exercise. The conversation was heard by the senses we call ears, but the information was not passed to our conscious mind by our filters. Think about your clothes, the crockpot, and the chair you are sitting in. The evidence that the filters have the ability to filter aspects of reality from your conscious experience is clear.

If believing this is too much of a shift, don't believe it. Just ask for more clarity. Ask yourself, could it be true? What sort of evidence might I see that will help me know? Where do I feel limited by limits that don't seem to apply to others? Can I shift those beliefs a little bit and just see what happens? Would that hurt anything? It would make me wrong but if I'm wrong do I want to cling to the old, wrong idea when adopting a new belief might serve me so much better? I don't have to believe this to play with the idea—to experiment a little bit.

That's not too much to ask, is it? It does not cost anything. No one even has to know. You can do every bit of it in the privacy of your own mind.

I can't prove any of this to you. But you can easily prove it to yourself; slight shifts in our beliefs literally change our world because our experience of reality is a personal interpretation. When you change a belief, the meaning you give to events shifts.

You may also be able to find examples in your own life.

Think about someone you know, or knew, who was struggling, perhaps with an addiction of some sort. We've all heard the stories. Think about them being offered a program would help them move on—a program where the benefits seem tremendous to you—yet they did not jump on the opportunity. In fact, they did not see the opportunity that was so clear to you.

They were in a state of hopelessness. They were filtering help out because they did not believe it would come.

Now you understand it better? Don't you?

Every thought you think receives an emotional response. Interpreted accurately, they will lead you directly to your dreams and goals.

The feeling we can reach for, no matter how we feel, is a feeling of relief.

Now, let's talk about guidance for a minute.

Our guidance is there for us all the time.

But how do we know?

I cannot prove it to you but you can prove it to yourself easily.

I can also show you science that shows we and all living things, have guidance.[106]

If you are frustrated, you are likely to notice something frustrating about your spouse, child, commute, boss, job, or world. Your filters essentially say, "Oh, she is feeling frustrated. She must want to feel that way. I will highlight this aspect of this situation because it will make her feel frustrated. I will highlight this aspect of this person because it will make her feel frustrated."

Your filter is not being mean when it does this. I am convinced it believes that if you are focusing in a way that makes you feel frustration and not using Right Responses to change your perception, that you want to feel frustrated.

I believe this because when you shift your perspective it does not continue showing you frustrating things. It begins showing you things that match your new emotional stance.

If you are in a state of appreciation, you will notice things you appreciate. I have managed myself into this state and maintain it on a fairly consistent basis. One huge difference I notice is my awareness of things I appreciate. For example, sitting on my deck, I will feel an impulse to look up just as the bright red Cardinal flies toward a tree. Once the bird is in the branches he is not visible but I looked up at the exact moment that allowed me to appreciate his plumage. It has become characteristic of me to interrupt conversations to say, "Look" as I point out something appreciable that has caught my attention. Yesterday it was a yellow finch that landed on my trellis. The bird was not there more than about 20 seconds, but I saw him land and take off. I was in the middle of a conversation with my fiancée as I was preparing to leave. I usually maintain eye contact when I am conversing but I glanced over to the other side of the driveway at exactly the right moment.

Few are those who see with their own eyes and feel with their own hearts.

Albert Einstein

I believe Einstein was referencing that we tend to believe what others think about us (and other things), even when it is not true.

Imagine how your relationships would change if what you notice first about your spouse, child, commute, boss, job, or world is something you personally find *pleasing.*

Your emotional stance does more than affect what you notice. It affects what you say. If you are in a state of appreciation, you are far more likely to offer compliments than criticism. What does that say about hurtful words someone may say to us?

Is it us? Or is it their current emotional stance?

Their emotional stance determines what aspects of you they focus on. Someone who is frustrated will notice something about you that can be frustrating. Someone who is angry will notice something about you that fuels their anger. Someone in a state of appreciation will notice something about you to appreciate. And for those of you who are wondering, it is possible for someone to live in those lower emotional states for decades. This is, unfortunately, a common question from students when I work on high schools.

The answer provides tremendous relief. If a child has been attempting to please an unhappy parent her entire life, she may be developing a belief about herself that will not serve her. She may be thinking she can't do anything right. But that is not true. The truth is her angry parent cannot perceive anything she does as right through a filter that is programmed to look for things that make the parent angry.

Do you want to see how absolutely wonderful your children are? You can't, not unless you program your filters to look for beauty in others. If you are looking at the world and calling it evil, you will not see the beauty in yourself or others. The way your filters are programmed affects your life in profound ways. There is nothing that is more important anyone can do than become consciously aware of how the filtering process affects their experience and begin adjusting the programming to serve their highest good.

Recognizing that if another person felt good he would find something nicer about you to focus on takes the sting from angry and bitter words.

Make up your own opinion about yourself. Do not accept what others tell you about yourself as true unless your guidance agrees. That means your heart sings when you hear the words. If you feel bad, that is your internal lie detector telling you the words are not truth—not your truth. From the other person's perspective, they may believe they are true. Arguing serves no purpose. Just know, in your heart and mind, that when the words sting it is your guidance telling you there is a perspective that will feel better to you. Then look for it or simply let it go as an untruth that does not have to distract you from whatever it is you are about. Do not give others the power to hurt you. Their words only have the power you give them.

Sometimes the nasty words come from a nasty person living in your mind. Someone who continually tells you what is wrong with you. If that person lives in your head, kick him or her out. You can develop a kinder and gentler voice in your head by refuting the nasty voice and reinforcing more positive attributes about yourself, to yourself, in the privacy of your own mind.

You do not need to feel bad to be motivated.

You can be motivated at the high ends by interest, passion, joy and feelings so good they are ineffable.

To summarize: More information than we can consciously manage is picked up by our senses in every moment. The filtering process between the raw data and information the conscious mind perceives uses our programming to decide what data reaches our conscious mind. In essence, our brain interprets reality in a way that proves our beliefs to us. The filtering process does not take into consideration whether the information that is filtered out would benefit our highest good. It does not care if we want the information. This is not about punishment—it is merely how it is programmed. I believe this is because the design is such that we are expected to understand how the filters work—that we are supposed to deliberately program the filters to serve our highest good.

I can tell you that for myself and thousands of others who have learned the techniques to re-program these filters, their lives have improved significantly. The improvements begin immediately and continue coming.

> *"Happiness is also a way of interpreting the world, since while it may be difficult to change the world, it is always possible to change the way we look at it."*
>
> *Matthieu Ricard*

Our beliefs create a powerful filter. Scientists know our beliefs are formed by about age 6. Almost no one deliberately changes their beliefs. The reason is that, because of the filters, once a belief is established it appears to be true. Our filters pass information that supports our beliefs to our conscious minds. Information that contradicts our beliefs is either not passed to our conscious minds or is interpreted to mean something consistent with our current beliefs.

Think about Semmelweis's hand washing recommendation. Before microscopes, the idea that we were surrounded by and covered with things too small for us to see would have gone against our beliefs and would have been frightening to contemplate. Even with his research showing a 31% decrease in the death rate, from 32% to 1%, the general population and even other physicians ridiculed him. They weren't stupid. The filters in their minds that did not pass information that conflicted with their beliefs to their minds and/or misinterpreted the information in a manner that was consistent with their beliefs.

Once a microscope was invented, revealing the presence of viruses, germs, bacteria and other microorganisms, hand washing became not only accepted, but mandated. They reference this shift in human ability to measure reality as if we "discovered" the organisms. In fact, that word, discovered, is telling. The microorganisms existed before the microscope but humans speak as if things do not exist until we perceive them, or discover them. In most instances, there is evidence that something exists before we measure it. The discovery is usually credited to the person who figures out how to measure it. The individual who knew there was something and recommended ways to benefit from it before it was measurable is often lost to history. We delay humanity's benefits by waiting until the ability to measure something is developed. I think we can be smarter than that. What do you think?

Chapter 13: Beliefs, Expectations, Emotional Stance, and Focus

Success or failure depends more upon attitude than upon capacity, successful men act as though they have accomplished or are enjoying something. Soon it becomes a reality. Act, look, feel successful, conduct yourself accordingly, and you will be amazed at the positive results.

William James

Beliefs are just thoughts an individual keeps thinking. In a global sense, some are valid and others are not. However, when an individual believes the thought, his life will demonstrate the truth of his belief to him. Our minds will show us evidence of our beliefs and will not show us evidence of things outside our beliefs.

Some of our beliefs support our highest good while others limit our ability to thrive.

In the 1980's movie "Rainman," Raymond (played by Dustin Hoffman) could accurately count the number of toothpicks dropped in a millisecond. The number was around two hundred and forty-three. This is an example of the information your brain receives in every moment. Most of our filters would not pass the count (243) to our conscious minds. This could be due to a belief that we cannot know the number without the physical act of counting. It could be due to a lack of focus in the way that would be required to pass the information on to our conscious mind.

The reason you can hear someone say your name in a loud room is because your filters are programmed to pay attention to your name. As a Mom, my filters are programmed to hear the word Mom, but only if the voice sounds like one of my daughters. If the voice is significantly different from my children's voices, I do not notice someone calling for their Mom when I am focused on something else.

As one's emotional state moves to higher zones, differences feel less relevant. There is research indicating that the way people tend to see people like them as "same" and people who differ from them as "other" lessens when positive emotions increase[107].

Believing that our brain shows us reality leads us to believe the information it passes to our conscious mind is an accurate reflection of reality.

Beliefs do not just hold people back. Those who developed empowering beliefs soar. Studying the beliefs of those who are thriving and compare theirs to your own can help an you identify beliefs you might like to adopt. *The Magic of Thinking Big,*[108] by David Schwartz is highly useful for this process.

Whether you believe you can, or you believe you can't, either way you're right. Which are you?

Henry Ford

The expectation filter plays a massive role in success. If an individual expects exceptional opportunities, he is far more likely to spot them. If he does not expect much, the opportunity could be right in front of him, and he will not recognize it. The brain will not pass information, which contradicts or exceeds expectations, to the conscious mind, even when the information is right in front of the person.

In my own career, I remember some of the deciding moments when I realized I could expand my goals. I remember giving a speech when I was just 21. There were two speakers that day; we were both being honored for obtaining a highly respected designation. The other speaker, a Vice President where I worked, had begun fulfilling the requirements for achievement of the designation before my birth. I gave a 7-minute speech with no notes to over 400 people, including all the executives. He read his in a monotone voice. I clearly remember realizing that if a Vice President could take more than 20 years to earn a designation I had earned in 23 months, and do such a poor job on the speech in comparison to my performance, that I could be a Vice President. It did not mean it would happen that day, but my personal perspective of my potential changed in that minute. My expectations for my life changed. When the opportunity came, I saw it clearly.

Our expectation plays a huge role in how we age. If we see a certain age as being old or anticipate ill health at that age, we are far more likely to experience that age in that way. When we change our perception of that age, our personal experience of it changes[109].

Regarding expectation, think of the children who do not thrive no matter the resources sent their way. Ask yourself, what is the expectation? Then, do all you can to increase the expectation if you are around any of those children. The potential of someone who lives without what is desired is even greater than that of someone who lives a mild life—once it is unleashed.

Influence of Expectation

Expectations greatly impact accomplishments. A bias toward optimism or pessimism influences assumptions individuals make about the future, as do people's past experiences. An experience in the past that resembles a current situation may cause the brain to interpret it as the same even if there are significant differences. One way to ensure one's expectations are serving the highest good is to think more deeply about why we view things the way we do. Emotional guidance is of great value in helping discern better ways to perceive our environment; the EGS contains more wisdom than the brain.[110]

There are also many examples of the way humans do not do things considered impossible but once one person accomplishes such a feat, whether it is learning to walk again after a spinal cord injury or running the first 4-minute mile, others who hear of it become able to do the same.

Our belief or lack of belief in our ability to accomplish something plays an important role in whether or not we succeed.

When we use what others have accomplished to determine what is possible, we limit ourselves to the successes of our predecessors. It is possible to use our EGS to determine what is possible for us. If we are ill should we think the thought, "There is a way for me to get better" and compare the emotional response to that to the emotional response to the thought "I am going to die."? The thought that there is a way for me to get better will feel better to anyone who has not decided they actually want to die (which does happen). If an individual has practiced using her guidance and trusts it, then the message will be clear that hope is not misplaced and there is a way. That belief opens up possibilities that do not exist when one believes it is hopeless.

Developing familiarity with one's own guidance system to the point where trust is developed can provide as much advantage as knowing someone else has accomplished our goal. It opens the possibility of not needing anyone else to do it first before we believe it is possible. Stories about walking after spinal cord injuries are a good example. When it was believed hopeless, it was unheard of for someone to recover the ability to walk. Today there are frequent stories. Some are the result of new techniques but one has to ask, would anyone have developed those techniques if they believed it was hopeless, or did having hope stimulate new research? How much of what we "can't" do is the result of a belief that we can't?

We want to control others, often because we have low expectations of them. Research has shown that our expectations influence the outcome[111].

Chapter 13: Beliefs, Expectations, Emotional Stance, and Focus

My favorite study is one where an elementary teacher was told that two of her incoming students were exceptionally bright. The person who advised her of this did not have firsthand knowledge—he was merely the messenger. The two students were actually performing very poorly.

At the end of the year, the two previously poorly performing students were performing exceptionally well. The study was one of the ones that said, "We observed this but we do not understand it so we need to do more research." However, in quantum physics they have discovered the mirror neurons[112], which explain how our expectations—high or low-influence others' behavior.

Students who could do better in the existing educational system are sometimes impeded by the strong and practiced low expectations of the teachers. Most teachers do not understand the impact of their own expectations on a student's performance. They are not taught how to cultivate positive expectations or why they are beneficial. Instead, prior outcomes for students from lower socioeconomic groups are used to establish the expectation—without realizing low expectations negatively impacted the outcome of the earlier students.

One of the best (and sadly somewhat common) examples of this is in a family where one person has been battling an addiction. The individual successfully completes rehabilitation and feels very confident about his future. Then he is back out in the world, amidst a family that is just waiting for him to backslide. The family did not go through the program with him so they anticipate another failure. If his intention and belief in his ability not to relapse is not greater than his family's expectation, the family's expectation will win.

Who wins when the expectations conflict? The one with the strongest belief wins. How do you counteract another's low expectations about you? Develop a stronger belief about who you are and where you're going than the ones held by those who see you as less successful.

Individuals in our society repeatedly define themselves based on how others perceive them. They allow others' low opinions to influence who they believe they are. Later in this book you'll see more clearly how another's opinion reflects who *they* are—not *who* you are.

Making conscious decisions about who you are and what you can accomplish is the best way to fulfill more of your personal potential.

Mirror neurons[113] do not require conversation or even body language. The mirror neurons sync to the stronger belief when we interact with one another. Have you ever ridden in an elevator with a complete stranger who seemed to think he was superior to you? Did you feel diminished as a result of the encounter? Was your self-esteem bruised?

If your answer is yes, strengthening your cohesion about who you are would benefit you.

We have the equipment to measure the syncing of the brains described by the term mirror neurons—but do not yet understand the mechanics behind the actual process. Research into biophotons is a promising area of research. Early work indicates biophotons are responsible for cellular communication in our own bodies—something earlier theories could not answer due to the instantaneous speed of the communication.

Our bodies quickly respond to stimuli, such as nervous perspiration the moment we are in a situation that causes us to be anxious or salivating the moment we see or smell something delicious. Chemical reactions in one cell triggering chemical reactions in adjacent cells does not account for the speed of our responses.

We should not wait until researchers reveal all the nuances of how mirror neurons work before we begin using what we do know to benefit one another. Seeing others for their potential rather than their current state would help them achieve more of their potential. This is true whether we ever speak a word about it to them.

What is "emotional stance"?

I have mentioned Emotional Stance (ES) before so let me clarify exactly what it is. I refer to ES in two distinct ways. One is the emotional stance in any given moment--how an individual feels in that moment in time. The other is their chronic emotional stance, a practiced emotional stance that an individual chronically returns to over time. It may be practiced deliberately or unconsciously, but everyone develops chronic emotional states. Individuals can change their chronic emotional state with deliberate effort, which is made easier by the use of their EGS. Both types of stances impact behavior and how the world is perceived.

Both our habitual and current emotional stance creates another filter. I manage my emotional stance to a place that feels good on a consistent basis, so my filter highlights information that feels good to me. It also dims negative aspects.

Emotional stance has more effect on behavior than the other filters. Emotional stance is tied directly to how empowered or disempowered we feel. Joy is a reflection of feeling very empowered. Depression reflects feeling very disempowered. Many undesired behaviors help an individual feel temporarily more empowered. If the individual understands how to use his or her EGS, there will be more socially approved methods of regaining a sense of empowerment. When individuals do not have that information, less desirable ways of feeling more empowered are chosen.

The first response to being in a lower emotional state than we are comfortable with is not usually crime. However, over time, especially if all the ways of increasing ones empowerment *perceptible to the individual* have been exhausted without success, crime becomes an acceptable method of regaining power (in the individual's mind).

Chapter 13: Beliefs, Expectations, Emotional Stance, and Focus

We naturally want greater degrees of empowerment. We can become comfortable in uncomfortable states (like the frog slowly boiling to death). An individual who has been depressed for a long time and unsuccessful in his attempts to regain power may eventually commit suicide or a murder/suicide or just murder. One of the reasons our society is so unsuccessful in helping individuals rise from depression is we reject aspects of the path from depression to more empowered states. Anger and revenge are more empowered than depression. We view those emotional states as more dangerous and discourage them. If it were generally understood that anger and revenge are no different than cities you have to drive through when they are along the route from Point A to the destination, Point B, we would do better.

You might have to stop for lunch but you do not have to buy a house in anger or revenge and take up residence indefinitely. When the path from depression to higher states is understood, assisting an individual quickly through the Hot Zone is not difficult.

Our society tends to see individuals who are moving into anger and revenge from depression as more troublesome (in those states) and push them back down to depression where they are easier to manage. We discourage anger, rather than guide the individual through anger to more empowered emotional states. This makes the path of anger appear blocked to the depressed individual, increasing the likelihood of criminal behavior being the next choice.

Chronic bad-feeling emotional stances are not cured through punishment. We cannot punish or guilt someone into better behavior. Individuals must be given the knowledge and skills to master their own emotional stance. Our guidance always points us toward better-feeling emotions. More importantly, it eliminates the sense that the only path to feeling better is one society abhors. In fact, after some experience, reaching the Hopeful Zone is easy because once you understand a tool that works, finding the feeling of hope is easier.

White-collar crime increases during economic declines. Underneath, it is often someone who was more afraid than they were in a better economy who commits the crime. Selling corporate secrets or client lists to competitors is not just a lack of ethics—it is fueled by fear. The fear comes from a mindset (belief) that the person has no control over her financial future and that it is in peril.

The employee who feels confident about his future will not commit the crime. Doing so would make the person feel less empowered. We act in the direction that will increase our sense of empowerment. This is true even when it does not appear to be the case to observers. If you could know, thought by thought, the way the individual perceives the decision; it would become clear that the words or actions were chosen because they felt more empowering.

When we are in lower emotional states, the contrast between our thoughts and our goals creates stress. When we change our thoughts in a direction that supports our dreams and goals, the stress decreases. If you practice paying attention to the emotional feedback from your thoughts for a while—the length depends on how attuned you are when you begin paying more attention—you can literally think a thought and feel the stress go up or down in your body, depending on which direction the thought takes you.

Emotional stance affects every relationship in our lives, from strangers on the road to our most intimate relationships in our homes. While the higher emotional states support close and loving relationships, the lower emotional states contribute to frequent friction and problems.

Each zone has a myriad of emotions within it. The separation is by the degree of empowerment felt while those emotions are being experienced.

Emotions are responses to thoughts and each thought elicits a new emotion. The emotion is the sensory guidance feedback systems response to the thought. Two consecutive thoughts may generate the same emotion or emotions so close to one another they cannot be differentiated, but the emotion changes in response to each thought. This can be easily shown using a guided meditation designed to move the emotions around. Changes in emotions are quickly recognized. Please see my website for a recording of this visualization which is listed in the back of the book.

Another thing to understand is that you have an emotional stance on every topic. When you hold an infant in your arms, you may immediately move to the top with feelings of love. When you hear of violence on the news you may immediately move to anger or fear. Even specific people you have not talked to or seen in years will have an emotional set point wherever it was when you last left it.

You can even have a different emotional stance for every topic. Find your set point on the EGS and then reach for the next higher emotion on that subject. You will not be able to move up more than 1 or 2 levels at one time, but you don't have to remain at a level any longer than it takes to become stable there before you can begin successfully moving up another level.

"Topic" must be very narrowly defined. Your relationship with your mother can be different from your relationship with your father. Your relationship with your mother on a specific subject, say money, can be different from your relationship with her on other topics such as gifts, food, shopping, clothes, career, marriage, or travel. The way you generally feel about your mother will have more to do with which topic you focus on when you think of her. If your mind automatically goes to the one troubled topic between you, you will experience the relationship as if you do not have a good relationship, even if there are dozens of other topics on which your relationship with her is good. If your mind tends to ignore the topic(s) where there is disagreement and focuses on those where harmony exists, you will feel you have a good relationship with her, even if one or more of the topics where there is dissention are areas of significant discord.

This example clearly demonstrates that our relationships with our mothers (and really anyone) are under our control as far as how we view it. If you decide to wait until your mother changes on the point(s) of discontent before you can be happy, you may wait forever. If you change your focus away from the areas where you disagree to the areas where there is harmony, you can feel better about your relationship right away.

At first, it requires a conscious effort to focus on different aspects of your relationship. This is only because your previous habit of thought created neural pathways in your mind that are easier for the neurons to travel than the new, more desired paths. The refocusing of your attention requires patience with yourself. If it is a topic you think about often, it will take about three months to shift your neural pathways. When you find the old perspective coming to your mind, recognize it is merely an old habit that has not yet been fully replaced with the new habit. Do not criticize yourself for the old habit not yet being gone. As soon as you recognize the thoughts, deliberately think about the thoughts you would rather focus on. This reinforces the new path.

When I listen to stories from people whose prior efforts failed to achieve the desired changes, this is where the failure most often occurred. It was not because the attempt to change was not working, but because their expectation and interpretation of how long it would take to change the habits of thought did not match their experience. They could not see how close they were getting to the goal and gave up, often within sight of the finish line. One of the main factors that contributed to giving up was the tendency to berate themselves for not yet achieving the goal.

Changing our thought processes requires kindness to oneself. Just making a conscious decision to change is a big deal. Give yourself credit for doing that and then allow time to assist you. I have deliberately made many changes to my thought processes. One in particular was extremely ingrained. I was much like Pavlov's dog when the subject came up. It was as if I carried a soapbox on my back and as soon as the subject came up, I would set the box down, climb on it, and begin spouting my beliefs about the topic to all who would listen. I had strong conviction that my beliefs were right. (They weren't.)

After my research convinced me that those beliefs were based on false premises, I decided to change them. I no longer believed them to be true. I would still find myself a few minutes into my tirade before my mind would engage. I remember the first time I realized what I was doing. I was back on my soapbox, spouting things I no longer believed, about five minutes into my typical spiel. I stopped talking, took a deep breath, and ended the conversation. Then I spent some time mentally reviewing the new beliefs about the subject. I felt appreciation that I now knew more and understood the truth.

The next time, I was only about five sentences into the old habit before I stopped myself. Soon, I would realize that I was going where I did not want to go in the first sentence. My EGS was helping because I had also been working on being more sensitive to the onset of negative emotions. I celebrated when I stopped myself at just the thought, before I uttered the words I no longer believed. The next time I thought about it, the thought was that it had been a few months since I had traveled that neuropathway. Now it has been years.

∞

Focus is the easiest significant filter to consciously direct, but it, too, has default modes. When one's focus is not responding to deliberate intentions, it uses its default settings, which differ because of many other factors.

Most people focus on whatever is in front of them. It can be the news channel where the negative emotions elicited are not recognized as a sign that watching it is not serving their highest good. It can be the latest fad or the hot new television show.

There are exceptions. Passionate interest in a topic will guide ones focus.

Unconsciously focusing on what we do not want ruins many relationships. Let's say a man went golfing with the guys on Saturday afternoon and had a five some in front of them, so they were unusually slow. He had told his wife he would be home at a certain time. Maybe they were going to see a movie, going to dinner, or she was cooking for him. He did not call her to let her know he would be late. Because she was looking forward to an activity that did not work out because he was delayed on the golf course, she feels upset. She is thinking about what she lost, the opportunity to see the movie, go to dinner, or that she took the time to fix dinner for him, and it was overcooked because he arrived late—it does not matter what it is. We are not talking about a big deal here. We are talking about something that could be perceived in many ways, but she is upset, so she focuses on his action rather than something that feels better to think about. Maybe she calls her best friend and tells her about it. She really gets a head of steam up about the perceived problem.

It is bad enough that she spent time feeling less emotionally good when she could have focused elsewhere and felt good the entire time. Doing so depresses her immune system during the time she is upset and increases the stress she experiences. She also spread the lack of joy by telling her girlfriend about her irritation. She probably said, "How irritated he made me," but the truth is that her perspective caused the irritation.

By placing the blame for her irritation on him, she has no power to fix it. She can be upset all she wants but if she is going to allow his lateness to upset her, she does not have control over how she feels. That is a disempowered perspective.

It can get worse. After the couple is all made up and happy with one another again, the friend, in a misguided attempt to be supportive, will say, "Has he done anything else that is irritating?" That just refocuses the unhappy wife's attention on the issue again. The focus filter will begin highlighting irritating things, instead of for reasons to love.

Your mind will point out what you focus on and ignore information you are not focused on. Once a member of a relationship begins looking for the unwanted they can't see desired behaviors, even when they are present. They have changed their perspective. They are no longer giving their partner the benefit of the doubt. The "back story" they begin assigning to the other's actions changes. The same actions that were once interpreted as loving may now be interpreted in a less pleasing way.

I often hear comments such as "I don't even know who he is any more" or "She's changed so much I am not sure she was ever the woman I thought I knew" and other similar remarks. Most people have no clue that their perception changed far more than the other person did. More importantly, they do not understand their own power to adjust their focus to a better-feeling place to put the relationship back on track. If they knew how simple it could be to get back on track, the divorce rate would plummet.

What could she have thought instead of being frustrated by his tardiness after his golf outing? She could have focused on being happy that he is able to go spend time with his friends. Leisure activities he enjoys make him happier, which makes him a better husband[114]. She could use the time to do something she enjoys. Even while she waited for him, she could:

- Read a book she enjoyed
- Call a friend
- Edit pictures
- Paint her nails
- Learn something new
- Spend time on a hobby
- Meditate
- Watch a movie
- Garden
- Listen to music

Can you think of other activities she could have chosen instead of becoming upset? Would she feel more empowered or less empowered if she chose to use the unexpected time to do something she enjoys? In the long run, is she letting him off the hook or will repeatedly choosing to do things that feel good make her life better?

Chapter 14: Coherent Thought

Quantum theory provides us with a striking illustration of the fact that we can fully understand a connection though we can only speak of it in images and parables.
Werner Heisenberg

In quantum physics, quantum coherence means that subatomic particles are able to cooperate. Subatomic waves, or particles, can communicate with each other because they are highly interlinked by bands of common electromagnetic fields. When the waves are in sync, they begin acting like one giant wave and one giant subatomic particle. Coherence creates the ability to communicate, like a highly sophisticated computer system. Popp's work[2] provided a better answer to how communication could occur instantaneously across a living system.

Scientists refer to live bodies as living systems. Cells of living systems, on average, undergo 100,000 chemical reactions per second in a process that occurs simultaneously across the body. Every second billions of chemical reactions of various types are occurring.

Herbert Fröhlich, of the University of Liverpool, was one of the first to introduce the idea that some sort of collective vibration is responsible for getting proteins to cooperate with each other and carry out instructions of DNA and cellular proteins. Waves (at the quantum level) synchronize activities for the living system.

Fritz-Albert Popp researched both healthy and unhealthy subjects, eventually concluding that good health was a state of perfect subatomic communication (coherence) and ill health was a state where communication breaks down. We are ill when our waves are out of sync.

In quantum physics, waves are encoders and carriers of information. When two waves are in phase (sync), and overlap each other (technically referred to as "interference") the combined amplitude of the waves is greater than the combined amplitude of the two waves; there is a compounding effect.

---

[2] Fritz-Albert Popp made the first extensive analysis of biophotons

Chapter 14: Coherent Thought

Resulting Wave

Wave 1

Wave 2

Constructive Interference: Amplifies the power

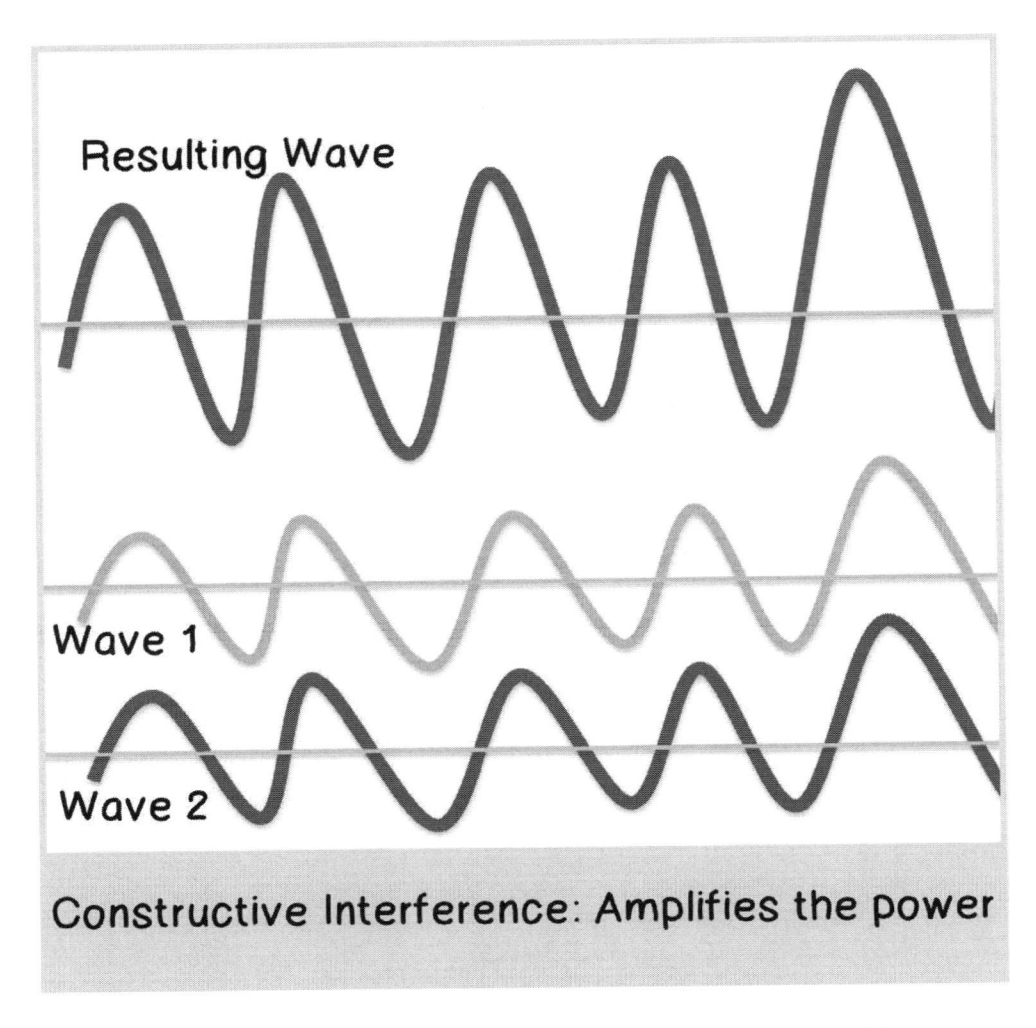

Imagine that a thought is wave 1 and a desire is wave 2. In this case, the waves are in sync (thoughts and desires are in sync). The individual in this situation would not have stress—waves in sync are not creating tension. The resulting outcome is positive. Popp found that individuals whose waves were sync were healthy.

This is consistent with research indicating that positivity and optimism confer significant health benefits, achieve greater success, experience fewer negative life events including fewer divorces, and generally experience lives with more desirable qualities.

Constructive interference could be represented by the desire "I want a job where I make enough to take good care of my family" amplified by the belief "I am well prepared to find a good job."

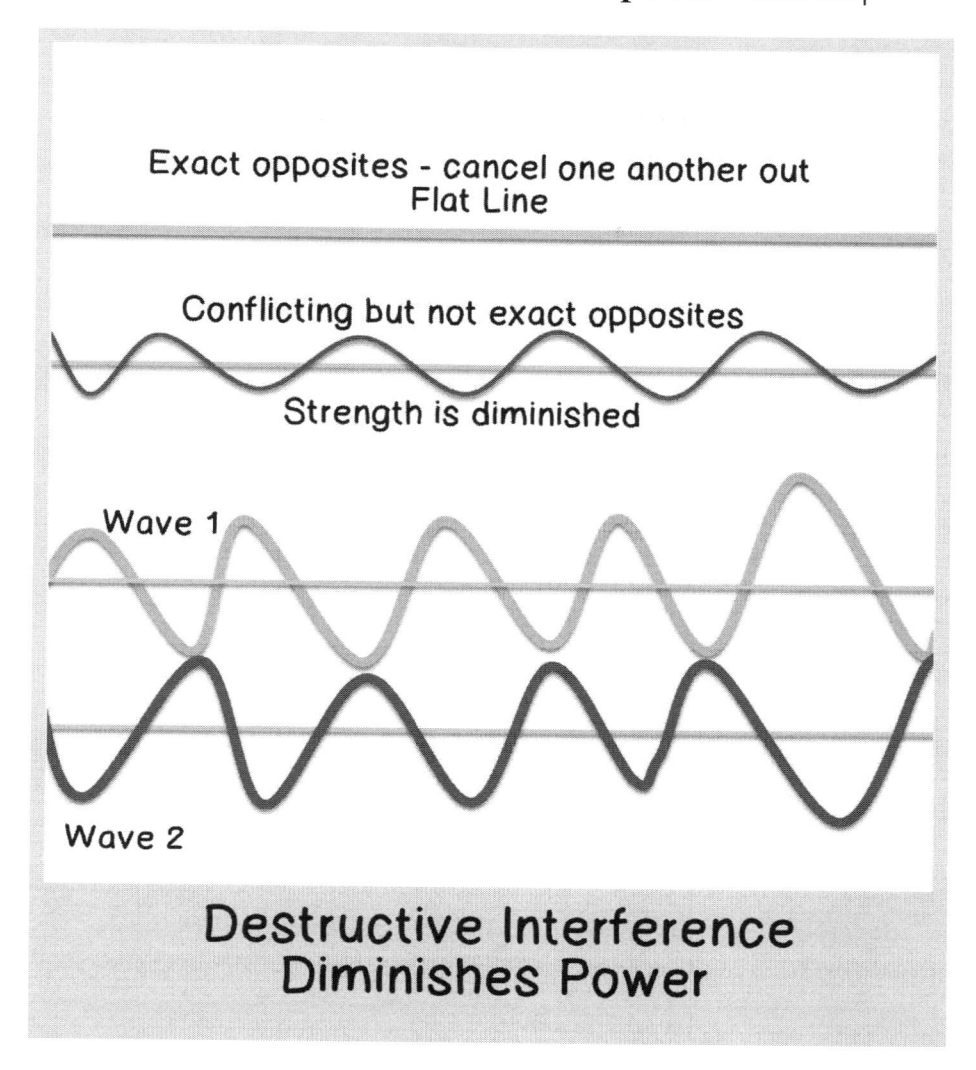

> **Exact opposites - cancel one another out**
> **Flat Line**
>
> **Conflicting but not exact opposites**
> **Strength is diminished**
>
> Wave 1
>
> Wave 2
>
> ## Destructive Interference Diminishes Power

The flat line is indicative of someone who wants something but whose belief is opposite the desire. For example, the desire "I want a job where I make enough to take good care of my family" contrasted with the belief "It is impossible to find a good job in this economy" would be a flat line.

The lower power wave could indicate the same desire combined with a less pessimistic (but still not positive) belief "It will take a long time to find a good job in this economy."

Can you feel how the conflict between the belief and the desire create tension or stress? This stress exists at the quantum level, which is why it is the root cause of ill health. When our thoughts are beliefs are in sync, the tension (stress) is reduced.

Although many people try, I have not found evidence of a way to pull back our desires. I have found ways to shift our beliefs to be more coherent with our desires. Increasing the constructive interference on the quantum level magnifies our success and our health.

Imagine that our thoughts are waves. A healthy, positively focused individual will have more coherent and positive thoughts. In other words, their thoughts will be consistently looking for solutions and believing they exist, their thoughts will reflect a belief that they will get through whatever hardship or turmoil they are surrounded by and be able to move forward. Or, if their life is going well, that it will continue to do so. Their waves are in sync, combining and amplifying one another. Communication with the body is consistent. The level of stress is low.

On the other hand, someone who is experiencing illness will want the same things, they will want to get through it and move on, they will want to believe things will turn out all right, but their negative bias will create destructive interference with the desires, thereby canceling out the thoughts of positive desires. Or, someone whose life is going well but who believes that it will not continue to do so creates destructive interference with continued wellbeing.

During my life time, we've shifted from a view of cellular communication that was the equivalent of a key being able to find its own keyhole to one that involves biophotons that move at the speed of light[115]. Science does not have all the answers yet, but this new direction seems to answer more questions. It is clear that a lot is going on that we have been unaware of because it occurs on a subtler level than our "five" senses. Imagine holding a meeting with hundreds of people in the room. You cannot hear the hum of the air conditioner. When you sit quietly in the same room when it is empty, you are able to discern the hum of the air conditioner.

In our normal state, input from our "five" senses is much like the meeting room with hundreds of people. The input from those senses is so clear and strong, the ability to perceive the subtler aspects of our environment is muted. I use quotes around "five" because we have far more than five senses. They could be more accurately categorized as, "The five loud senses." We are already aware that when one of the five loud senses is muted, as in someone who is deaf or blind, the perceptual ability of the remaining senses increases.

Three examples of thoughts and their coherence, or lack thereof , are shown below. The first example is of someone who lacks resilience and is in a low emotional state. Their thoughts are coherent and therefore amplified but they are coherent in a very negative way, causing a downward spiral.

Thoughts	Direction
I can't believe this is falling apart. Nothing ever works out for me.	↓
Every time I think something is finally working out it crashes.	↓
I can't remember the last time something worked out really well for me.	↓
I might as well stop trying. It never works out for me.	↓
I must be cursed. What is the point?	↓
I don't know what to do. I can't do anything well.	↓
Life is awful and then you die.	↓

In the next example, the random and unfocused thoughts of someone whose thoughts are inconsistent cancel one another out. The person has some positive thoughts, but not enough to cause thriving. If the thoughts continue to be more negative than positive, a downward spiral is a possibility.

Thoughts	Direction
I really hope this will turn out OK (thought without any real feeling of hope)	↓
Sometimes things turn out OK	↑
Maybe my brother will help me out (hopeful but no real faith)	↗
Bad things happen in three's; what is next?	↓
At least I have people in my life who will always love me no matter what	↑
I hope Joe never hears about this; he will never let me live it down	↙
Every time I think things are going well something bad happens	↓

Deliberately choosing to focus on better feeling thoughts could turn the situation around and create the far more desirable upward spiral. Most people's thought patterns are more like this second example. If they understood the importance of focusing on what they want with positive expectation, they would make a greater effort to increase thoughts that would benefit them.

This is at the root of why businesses have taught goal setting and other techniques that have proven successful. The techniques create greater coherence and amplify their ability to achieve them.

In this third example, of thoughts from a positively focused and optimistic mindset, the coherence of thoughts that support the individual's underlying desires increase wellbeing in all areas of life where this thought pattern is present.

Thoughts	Direction
Every time I think something bad has happened to me it turns out to be good when I get a clearer view of it	↑
I wonder what the silver lining will be here?	↑
I know there is a solution. There always is. I wonder what it is.	↑
Things always work out well for me. I don't have to know the ending to know this will work out well, too.	↑
I wonder what new things I will learn because of this?	↑
It is fun to solve problems.	↗
I have lots of people who will help me if I need help.	↑

Comparing the above examples of thoughts, the scattered, powerless nature of the middle example and the greater power and cohesion in the first and third examples can be felt.

On the quantum level, we understand that as these coherent thoughts overlay one another, the combined strength is amplified because they are coherent. The first and last examples are indicative of individuals whose situations are changing because their coherent thoughts have amplified power. Unfortunately, for the individual thinking the thoughts with a strong negative bias in the first example, they are moving in the opposite of the direction they want to move. The middle example, representing a more common thought-pattern, characteristic of a person who seems to be moving in circles or chasing their own tail, so to speak. They move around a little bit but often end up back where they began.

Sometimes an event in one's life causes a temporary decrease in her perception of worthiness. This results in a decrease in wellbeing in areas that may have previously evinced a strong coherent pattern of thought toward their desires.

In essence, the emotional stance decreases. For individuals who live in the public eye, such as Donald Trump and Tiger Woods, it is possible to see the dip in their success while the emotional stance is lower. Eventually, they return to their original chronic stance. It is possible to shorten the duration of the downturns using the techniques outlined in this book. The same dips occur in private lives. If you think about your own life, you will see evidence of this.

The discussion about set points on topics applies here as well. Someone can have cohesive positive thoughts about one area of life and destructive interference in another area of life. Some factors create spillover into many areas of life. Self-esteem, or worthiness, is one of the areas that will have an effect across the board. Other factors may only effect one aspect of life or an even narrower topic, such as a single relationship or goal.

Your EGS will guide you toward greater positive coherence.

Write one of your goals or desires at the top of the blank chart below. Use the chart to record your own thoughts. Add arrows to indicate the whether your thought patterns are consistent or inconsistent with your goal. Nuances do matter. "I can" is not equal to "I think I can," use your EGS to feel for the difference between the two thoughts.

If your thoughts do not currently support your goals, use the processes in Chapter 17 to shift your thoughts to ones that support your goals. A separate chart for each topic can be beneficial. However, the goal is not to complete a lot of charts. The goal is to feel how the emotional discord feels and adjust your perception to one that feels better.

Thoughts	Direction

Do you need some help coming with idea for your topics? Do you have a health condition that is not as good as what you would like it to be? Use that to see if your thoughts are in alignment with recovery.

If you enjoy good health, you can use the way you feel when you are ill—such as when it feels like a cold is starting. Another alternative is to think about how you think about an illness someone you care about is experiencing. Remember, the mirror neurons and the influence of expectation.

Another way to use the chart is to ask your friends about things you say on a regular basis. One example is "I can gain weight just from smelling the cakes in the bakery."

Because our society currently operates as if the quantum level does not exist or matter, there are many common beliefs and phrases that do not serve our highest good. At first, I did not think such thought could really matter. However, after consistently feeling for how different thoughts felt, I began to feel the discord of unsupportive thoughts in a stronger way. When that happened, I shifted my mindset away from unsupportive thoughts and my results changed.

Here are some more examples of common unproductive expressions:

- *A good man is hard to find.*
- *I always choose the slowest line at the checkout counter.*
- *I can never (fill in the blank). i.e. find my keys*
- *I always (fill in the blank). i.e. anything you don't want*
- *Nothing good lasts forever.*
- *I am always a day late and a dollar short.*
- *He does not respect me.*
- *I can't (fill in the blank). i.e. anything you want to do*
- *(fill in the blank) is too expensive for me to do.*
- *It's a once in a lifetime experience. (unless you only want to do it once)*

Can you think of expressions you think or say that may be creating destructive interference with your ability to achieve your goals?

Chapter 15: Happiness Defined

When I was 5 years old, my mother always told me that happiness was the key to life. When I went to school, they asked me what I wanted to be when I grew up. I wrote down 'happy'. They told me I didn't understand the assignment, and I told them they didn't understand life.

John Lennon

    As the research about happiness has grown, the pursuit of happiness has received some criticism in research that, on the surface, seemed to indicate contra-findings. I reviewed much of that research and found the reason for their results in their details. For example, researching individuals who are focused on "finding happiness" does not provide insight into the benefits of happiness. The study participants were unaware of their emotional guidance and did not have knowledge or tools to facilitate being happy. They were less happy than they would have been without a focus on a goal they did not know how to attain.

    This research does not speak to any contra-indications about happiness. It speaks to the great need humanity has for tools and knowledge that allow individuals to experience positive emotions quickly and easily. The search, combined with their lack of knowledge and skills about how to attain happiness, led to a diminishing belief in their ability to achieve happiness. As a result, they felt less empowered. Happiness does not require pursuit. It does not require a search, but the proper knowledge and skills. Fortunately, we now know the knowledge and skills that facilitate happiness. We also know that the processes are simple to understand. Happiness is within everyone's reach.

    The findings that individuals who were focused on the goal of happiness but did not know how to achieve it and therefore were more stressed and not as happy would be anticipated based on the EGS. The lack of knowledge about how to be happy would cause a lower emotional state and higher stress—thus decreasing happiness.

    A more helpful study would gather data about an individual's current level of positivity, provide the knowledge and skills to increase happiness, and then take new measurements about the level of positivity. A study that followed the participants over time, looking at not only increased positivity but also health status would be of the greatest benefit to humanity.

When I introduced the idea that happiness and chronic stress are two ends of the same continuum, I mentioned that stress and happiness being opposites is not my definition of happiness. To me, this is a trait, but not the definition of stress and happiness. Many situations cause individuals to feel positive emotions, temporarily. There is nothing wrong with enjoying things that make us happy, but using them as the basis for being happy sets us up for failure.

The Chapter 18 discusses many of the things that hold an individual back from being happy. Basing happiness on outer conditions is the way most of humanity currently approaches the subject. Some common, conditional happiness delaying techniques include:

"I'll be happy when I find the person I want to marry."
"I'll be happy when I get that promotion."
"I'll be happy when I get to go _____ on vacation."
"I'll be happy when I have a baby."
"I'll be happy when I retire."
"I'll be happy when my children are grown."
"I'll be happy when I lose weight."

Unfortunately, outer focused criteria for happiness do not contribute to long-term sustainable happiness without negative side effects. Also, individuals who delay happiness using excuses like the above criteria do not know how to be happy so when the stated goal is achieved, another reason to delay happiness is typically substituted.

Here are the facts that negate the above delaying tactics:
- Happy people are more likely to marry and stay married. Happiness increases the ability to attract a desirable mate.
- Happiness is a precursor to success. Individuals who are more positively focused enjoy more careers that are successful.
- Many people go on vacation and bring their unhappy selves with them; forgoing much of the joy they could have on their journey.
- Stress (lack of happiness) poses several risk factors for individuals who want to have a baby. A stressed woman has more difficulty conceiving. Once conception occurs, a stressed woman's child has a higher risk of behavioral and sleep problems, asthma, and if she is depressed, the child's risk of depression increases. Even a depressed Father is linked to higher incidence of depression in the child[116]. The marriage of a happy couple provides the child with a more stable environment.
- By the time some people retire, they have been practicing unhappiness for a great many years. The habit of unhappiness is

entrenched. While someone who really did not enjoy their profession will feel better than they did while working, there is a difference between feeling better and being happy. Also, the benefits of happiness (better health, lower risk of every disease studied, better immune system functioning, increased cognitive abilities, better relationships, more successful careers, and more) are so significant, why would anyone wait until the last quarter of their life to enjoy the benefits?

- Waiting until the children are grown to be happier results in your teaching your children that happiness is not a priority. It also means you will not be as good of a parent as you could be. My children would tell you there is a significant difference in my parenting once I learned how to be happy in a sustainable way. It is a positive improvement. In many ways I wish I had known what I now know throughout their childhoods because I know I would have been a better parent.
- Being happy facilitates healthy weight management. As outlined in Chapter 5, the old paradigm of calories in equaling calories out has been overturned. Stress (which is essentially lack of happiness) causes the body to fight against your efforts to eat nutritiously and maintain the ideal body weight.

Basing our happiness on anything outside of ourselves brings the potential for adverse side effects. There is always the possibility that we will not be able to participate, or that someone we cannot control will disappoint us. I submit that true happiness requires greater stability and less reliance on outer, uncontrollable factors. One reason I insist on this definition of happiness is it is the only one in which the individual is empowered to choose happiness.

Sustainable Happiness Defined

The state of happiness does not require a constant state of bliss. It is a deep sense of inner stability, peace, well-being, and vitality that is consistent and sustainable. Awareness that one possesses the knowledge and skills to return to a happy state, even when not in that state, is a critical component of sustainable happiness.

With outer, uncontrollable factors, results are inconsistent. What made an individual feel joy at one time could have no impact or even a negative one at another time.

For example, when I was 18, a Monday – Friday job paying $400 a month made me feel great joy. That same job today would be terribly upsetting. Even if the wages were adjusted for inflation, it would still be far below my expectations.

Our goals are ever changing. Movement from wherever we are in the direction we wish to go—whether that movement is in thought or deed—feels good. Movement away from our goals—whether in thought or deed—feels bad.

One more thing humanity does on a widespread scale is judge whether another's circumstances are good based on their own desires. Each of us has a different perspective and desires that are uniquely our own. Our guidance considers our unique desires. The individual who wants to be a teacher is guided toward being a teacher, and the individual who wants to be an accountant is guided toward his goal. We feel good when we are moving toward our own goals.

If, when I was hired for the Monday-Friday job when I was 18, someone had begun pointing out to me how much less than many others I was making, or other aspects of my achievement they viewed as less than wonderful—based on their goals—it would have diminished my joy. At a point in life like that, excitement over one's first job that is perceived as the first step of a career, diminishing the achievement could diminish the motivation to be successful. Lower intrinsic motivation would result in lower success. Less success equates to less positive feedback. This creates a circle where intrinsic motivation declines, resulting in even less success.

> True happiness comes from positive movement towards our goals.

Some of us have family members who are experts at making us unhappy with our circumstances. We might be excited about movement in the direction we want to go and they immediately look for flaws in what we have achieved and point them out to us. They are comparing our achievement to their goals. We feel deflated by those encounters. If you have someone like that in your family or at work, it is often best not to share your excitement with him or her—so they do not go into their deflation routine. Give them the facts and share your excitement only with those who are supportive.

Positivity

As scientists study the subject of positivity, they also attempt to define it. In some instances, happiness is measured by a small action that creates a better emotion temporarily. This research demonstrates that the more positive emotion is good for the individual feeling it and also for those she interacts with, including strangers.

Researchers are using numerous terms to describe happiness including positivity, optimism, and General Wellbeing (GWB).

It does feel great to experience something that causes a temporary lifting of one's mood. The difference between a temporarily uplifted mood caused by something outside of ourselves, over which we have no real control, and deliberately adjusting our perspective to feel better without any reliance on the outer situation is like the difference between a baby who has learned to crawl and a world-class Olympic decathlon gold medalist.

The recent focus on happiness has received some backlash from some researchers. One common criticism of positivity is the belief that negative emotions are being repressed. This is not based on empirical evidence. In fact, in *Positivity*, Barbara L. Fredrickson, Ph. D. states, "On the contrary, resilience is marked by exquisite emotional agility."

There have been publications arguing that anxiety is good for us. They are right that we should feel anxiety—anxiety, like any other emotion—is communication. We should feel anxiety for 60 seconds or less, just long enough to assure ourselves that a solution is possible. We don't have to solve the problem—just the knowledge (which our EGS will affirm) that the problem is solvable—reduces anxiety. Reducing anxiety increases our cognitive abilities. Believing a solution is available primes our mind to be ready when information that leads to a solution comes into our awareness. I'm serious about the sixty seconds. In fact, for someone who has been utilizing her guidance consistently for a few years, sixty seconds may be longer than necessary. Solutions and the belief that solutions exist creates intrinsic motivation.

Some arguments have been put forth that positive emotions are not always good because anxiety can be a call to action. The goal is not to remain always joyful and carefree. The goal is to know that no matter what happens an individual knows how to return to being joyful. The accomplishment of a goal is not necessary to feel happy. Just progress toward the goal will bring emotional relief. When we feel anxiety, we should recognize it for what it is, emotional guidance, and then take appropriate action. Once appropriate actions begin, we can feel immeasurably better knowing that we are moving in the right direction. Their emotional response will give them this feedback.

The "call to action" resulting from anxiety pales in comparison to the "call to action" from passionate interest. The anxious individual does not dream the big dream. The anxious call is much further down on Manslow's Hierarchy of Needs. Typically, anxiety involves moving away from something undesired. Essentially, retreat. Passionate interest, on the other hand, is a movement toward something bigger than oneself that increases energy and motivation.

Optimists and pessimists are both often adamant about the correctness of their stance. Looking deeper, we find that they are both right because of the impact of expectation on outcome.

Examined more deeply, it becomes clear that positive expectation results in more desirable outcomes:

> *"People who regard themselves as highly efficacious act, think, and feel differently from those who perceive themselves as inefficacious. They produce their own future, rather than simple foretell it."*[117]

Chapter 16: Chronic Stress

The mind can go either direction under stress—toward positive or toward negative: on or off. Think of it as a spectrum whose extremes are unconsciousness at the negative end and hyperconsciousness at the positive end. The way the mind will lean under stress is strongly influenced by training.
Frank Herbert

In Chapters 1 – 8, evidence that stress is perhaps the most significant underlying cause of many illnesses, diseases, and undesired life events was introduced. Chapters 9 – 15 were designed to broaden the perspective about stress and its roots to create an environment receptive to new ideas about how to prevent illness.

This chapter brings it all together and takes the root cause of illness deeper, illustrating that individual mindsets determine the level of stress experienced by each individual. Circumstances do not dictate the level of stress. This is one of the most exhilarating aspects of human thriving, each of us has far more control over our life experience than we typically use.

Mindset = level of stress
Level of stress = level of enjoyment (or suffering)
Level of stress = higher or lower immune function
Immune function (coherence[3]) = health
Reliable tool to facilitate supportive mindsets = EGS

I won't go as far as to say stress causes all illness. I will say that if we apply the tools described herein broadly, the incidence of illness, and

---

[3] All the pieces of the puzzle are not yet known, but enough is known to be sure that coherence of thought enhances physical and mental wellbeing.

especially chronic debilitating illnesses, will be greatly diminished. This will solve the global healthcare crisis from expensive chronic illnesses. By eliminating the illnesses that strong stress management skills can prevent, the currently scattered resources can focus on any remaining unresolved problems.

Research has shown that positivity and optimism increase life expectancy by 10.7 years and increase healthy years of life by 18 years because the debilitating end of life diseases come much closer to death in positively focused individuals. The meta-analysis from Harvard showed positivity decreased the risk of developing heart disease by 50%.

We will not know the full effect until we implement these ideas. It is my most fervent desire that we move beyond the Galileo Effect and not wait until every nuance of how it could be so beneficial is proven before we adopt the changes that enable humanity to benefit from what we do know.

∞

Many people intellectually acknowledge how we perceive events in our lives determines how we feel about them. This is so obvious, it is difficult to miss. But deliberately changing our perspective so that we feel better is rare.

It is rare because we are taught to take action—the worse the perceived situation, the faster we should take action—so goes conventional "wisdom." This is how most of us are taught to respond to situations.

Action is not the first step. Finding the best possible perspective we can in the moment is the first step. This is true in every situation, even emergencies, which is why pre-paving your neural pathways to a positive focus is so critical to your ability to thrive. In the mindsets and emergencies section of this chapter, a fictional character experiencing an unexpected emergency demonstrates the effect of different mindsets on the actions and effectiveness of actions taken.

The impact of thought on subsequent action is not given its due in modern society. There is a common perception that adjusting thought patterns takes a long time and great contemplation. With practice, unproductive thoughts can be identified and adjusted quickly. A bystander might not even notice any hesitation, but the individual who adjusts the unproductive thought will receive immediate benefits. Adjusting thought results in better mental decisions, which ultimately lead to more success than could have been achieved with what I will term inferior thinking.

Let me pause here and mention that the label "inferior" thinking is not intended, in any way, to judge the individual thinking in that way. Everyone can learn how to adjust mental processes so that the conclusions reached support greater success. Inferior refers to the results achieved as the result of the thinking. Most individuals today have not been taught how to do this and have been taught myths that make the way they operate on auto-pilot seem like all they can do. It is not all they can do. The only difference between inferior thinking and thriving thinking is a little knowledge and some skills that even a child can learn.

Today, "inferior" thinking is widely accepted, within certain bounds set by society. This may be the greatest "Pay it forward" opportunity the world will ever see. As understanding that the underlying thought processes can be adjusted, we can help one another—not by telling others how to think or what to think—but by asking them questions such as, "Is there a perspective that would feel better about this?" or "Is there another way to perceive this situation?"

Or, for those who fully understand the importance of adjusting the mental attitude first, a gentle reminder like my fiancée has been known to give me, "Are you using old-fashioned thinking?" Once someone recognizes the importance of adjusting ones thoughts first, a gentle reminder like that is all it takes to help us recognize when old habits are still affecting our thoughts.

That brings up another important point. Many people have attempted some form of change in their thoughts. The "think positive" movement has been around a very long time. I've read many of the books. What they lacked is the "How." How do people change thinking processes to be more positive?

One of the very first things that is important for many individuals is to begin the process of ceasing their personal attacks on themselves. Most of us have been taught to be extremely self-critical. Self-criticism is not necessary for growth. In fact, it slows growth by creating doubts, lowers our energy level, makes us hesitate to reach for our goals, hinders our achievements, and creates chronic stress.

It does not matter if someone is a smoker, addicted to substances, not nice to others, practicing unhealthy habits, or any other habit they wish to improve—beating up on oneself does not help the solution happen faster. One reason is in order to achieve our goals we have to believe we can achieve them. Let's take the worst of the lot—not being nice to others. This can be anything from rude to criminal behaviors. The people who are beating themselves up already wants to change. If they did not want to change, they would not be beating themselves up.

It is not a function of good and evil people. It is a function of emotional stance, duration, and severity. For example, an act of violence done when suddenly discovering your spouse is unfaithful would be considered a severe change in emotional state. Someone who is bullied or abused repeatedly is an example of a sustained low emotional stance. Someone who experiences a sudden disappointment while overtired may react in temporary anger, but is less likely to become violent than someone who has been in a sustained low emotional state.—whereas someone who is habitually angry may allow the anger to linger or the situation to escalate to a larger problem than a "reasonable" person.

If you are beating yourself up for something you did in the past, you are different from the person who did the thing you are unhappy about having done. In essence, you are beating yourself up for who you used to be. If you were still that person, the prior decision would still make sense to you. You have learned something since that decision, or improved your emotional stance. In either case, you are not the identical person who made the decision.

I liken it to the following scenario. You wrote a rough draft of a book, then you read some books on grammar and storytelling, and maybe you hired someone to edit the book. Based on the changes recommended, you learned how to write better. You re-write the book, incorporating what you have learned, and you want to save it with the file name you used on the rough draft. You click "Save as" and try to save the file using the same file name. The computer says, "Version xx.1 already exists, replace?" Beating yourself up is like saying "Before I overwrite the original file, I have to find all the errors in the old one and tell everyone about them. I need to document the things I did wrong in the rough draft before I save the improved file on top of it."

That path just delays the creation of the improved version. You could be moving forward toward your goals, which is a less stressful activity than self-criticism. You do not need to go back and find every error you made in the original version because you are an improved version. You've learned more about grammar, about how to write a good story (in this analogy). Going back and figuring out where you weren't as good in the past as you are now is not productive. You could spend that time making even more improvements to the future version of you. Or you could spend that time just having fun. Anything you do instead of self-criticism be more productive for you. Just overwrite the old you with the new and move on.

It is possible to feel in harmony with something better when surrounded by chaos.

Being Positive or Positive Thinking

There is a distinct difference between the decision to be more positive and the achievement of the goal. To me, it appears as if we thought just informing people that thinking positive was desirable was sufficient to make the change. In fact, this has created a great deal of harm—because people feel guilty or feel that they failed when it did not work.

For example, The Center for Disease Control and Prevention (CDC) recommends:[118]

> "Most importantly, don't sweat the small stuff! Try to pick a few really important things and let the rest slide — getting worked up over every little thing will only increase your stress. So, toughen up and don't let stressful situations get to you! Remember, you're not alone — everyone has stresses in their lives...it's up to you to choose how to deal with them."

This does not provide any information about "how" to actually "let it go" which is critical to actually being able to let it go as opposed to suppressing the emotion—which is harmful to mental and physical health. In fact, the "toughen up" language implies a form of suppression—ignoring the negative emotion caused by the thing(s) that are bothering one—rather than addressing the perception (which leads to the emotions) in a straightforward manner.

It is critical that sources that should be trustworthy, such as the CDC, stop promoting advice that does not go far enough and that is easily interpreted to suggest unhealthy practices –such as suppressing emotions. Dr. David Spiegel, commenting on research that found women who perceive life events as stressful have shorter disease-free intervals in relationship to breast cancer when compared to women who perceive the events as lower in stress, was quoted by the National Institute of Health:[119]

> "Our research has shown that people do better in the aftermath of traumatic stress if they deal with it directly. Facing, rather than fleeing it, is important. We have conducted support groups for more than 30 years, and found that dealing with traumatic and very stressful experiences is much healthier. In other words, don't suppress your emotions."

One of the key points of TRUE Prevention is that two people can experience the same type of life event with one perceiving it as very stressful while another manages the stress so that the event is not a big, hairy deal. It is not about controlling whether or not bad things happen in our lives because not all relationships are harmonious throughout life, some people participate in dangerous occupations, others experience violence or verbal abuse, people we love die before we do, and other events we do not desire occur. But how we perceive them, how much stress our bodies feel as a result, is within our control. Stress management skills can greatly reduce the stress we feel from such situations, which will have a significant difference on our health, mental well-being, relationships, and success in life.

Properly setting expectations is critical to success. Becoming more positively focused occurs on a couple of parallel continuums. There is the intellectual decision, "I want to be more positively focused." This is the first step in the process but without more, it is not productive.

I think what trips most people up is that the action steps in becoming more positively focused are mostly mental. Yes, there are physical action steps that help—some of those have been taught. In fact, most teachers focus exclusively on physical steps.

Some examples of physical steps include:

- Gratitude journals
- Mindfulness
- Positive affirmations
- Helping others
- Being in nature
- Exercise
- Meditation
- Give someone a compliment
- Learn something new
- Compare yourself to someone who is worse off
- Drink less caffeine
- Smile
- Eat more nutritiously
- Listen to relaxing music
- Eat dark chocolate
- Drink a glass of red wine
- Take a bath
- Take a walk
- Get a massage

All but two of the above steps can be counter-productive if not accompanied by a beneficial mental attitude. In the discussion of processes in the next chapter, I elaborate on the mental attitude aspect. Meditation and mindfulness are not, to my knowledge, counter-productive. While meditation and mindfulness by themselves do not achieve the results that are possible with deliberate adjustment of perspective, both are powerful methods of improving life and can create significant improvements. Using meditation in conjunction with Right Responses provides individuals with greater mental strength.

All of the other commonly suggested methods of feeling better have too many underlying variables—they work for some people and not for others. They work for people some of the time, but not always. They are saturated with exceptions. I want the realization to become automatic that when there are many exceptions, it means we are treating a symptom, not the root cause[4].

The root cause reason that someone is feeling bad is not addressed by the common recommendations. The recommendations often create a temporary lifting of mood. There is nothing wrong with using them when

---

[4] The Parsimony Principle in science tells us that the simplest explanation, the one with the least numbers of exceptions, is probably the most accurate.

they help, but the underlying reason the person felt bad to begin with is not addressed or changed by them.

Just as a Band-Aid does not heal the cut, those methods do not heal. Both physical and emotional well-being depends on our state of mind. We have shrouded the mind in secrecy. As a group, humans tend not to share their underlying thoughts with others. We function very superficially. We have regulated such discussions to psychiatrists and psychologists—a common belief exists that professionals must be involved if we want to change our thought processes.

Let's look at those professionals for a moment. Until recently, none of them studied human thriving. The focus of their education was on what could go wrong in human thinking. Labels were created and applied to form "clinical diagnoses." Some of these diagnoses were curable and others incurable. A great deal of effort and dialogue over the best method of curing the labels continues to occur.

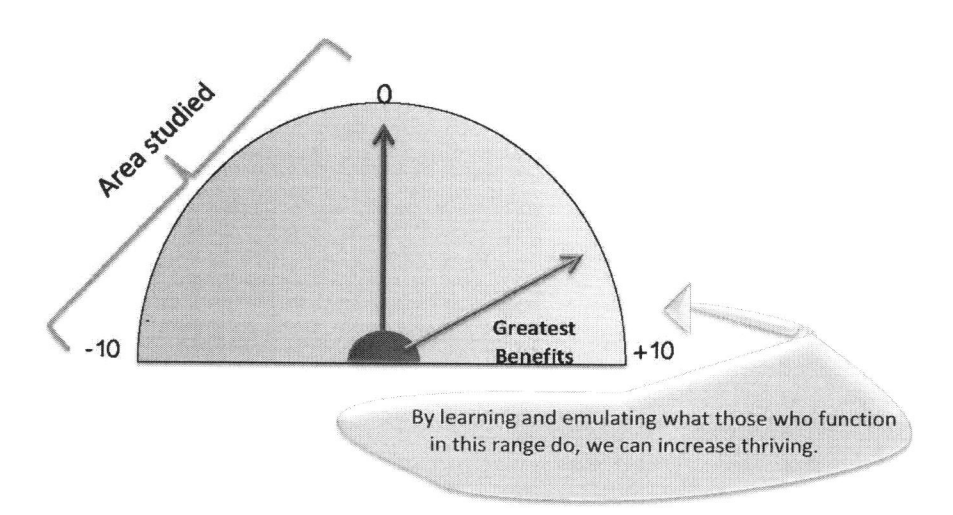

Area studied: -10 to 0. Greatest Benefits: toward +10. By learning and emulating what those who function in this range do, we can increase thriving.

On this scale, -10 equates to severe depression, +10 equates to joy, enthusiasm, love, and appreciation. Zero is above depression but it is a long way below happiness. Dr. Martin E.P. Seligman introduced the field of Positive Psychology when he was President of the American Psychological Association in 1998.

Prior to that, the mental health community defined individuals as "well" when they were at zero. Their curriculums of psychologists and psychiatrists focused on conditions found between -10 and 0. Insurance typically did not provide much in the way of mental health benefits and someone above zero is considered not in need of mental health benefits.

Like other areas of medicine, in mental health we studied the ill in our attempts to discover the cure. The solution is not found in the ill. It is found in those who are well. By studying what makes a person thrive, we learn what individuals who are ill need to do to achieve similar results.

This is not intended as criticism of mental health professionals or the profession itself. It is historical fact, which contributed to the public perception that mental health work had to be done by professionals.

Vast progress is rapidly being made in understanding the benefits of a positive mental attitude. The world will not benefit fully from this new knowledge until our attitude about mental health changes. Great beneficial changes are possible for anyone who cultivates within himself or herself a positive mental attitude.

Understanding that feeling good is healthy for you and struggling under negative emotions leads to both physical and mental illness does not require time on a therapists' couch. Understanding how filters affect your perception of reality does not require therapy. Understanding how to adjust your filters is guided by your emotional guidance system, which gives you immediate feedback in response to every thought you think. If it feels better, it is better for you. If it feels worse, it is worse for you.

The one caveat is that someone who is depressed moves through anger and revenge on their way to joy. Don't take physical action in the hot zone. Use imagery to move up. If you think you might act while in that zone, get help.

No action is required to feel better.

If you need to imagine doing things to someone to help you move past the powerlessness you feel from having been a victim, imagine things you can't really do. For example, imagine you have a space ship and you somehow take them aboard and strand them on Pluto or some other planet. You'll feel better, but you won't be tempted to act on the idea.

That the path to joy from depression travels through anger and revenge is one reason so many get stuck in depression. When we're depressed we're not much fun but we are a whole lot less trouble than someone who is anger or vengeful—at least until we have had all we're going to take and move up in an out of control manner. There is no reason to stay depressed long enough to bottle up that much hurt and pain.

The journey from depression to above anger and revenge can be done in less than an hour with a little practice. You'll feel better in the long run if you travel through the hot zone in your mind without physically going there. Don't imagine scenario's you might or could actually do. You have an imagination—use it. Be creative. If you find yourself fixating on something that you begin thinking you need to do, stop. Re-focus on something else or ask for help.

Remember that actions you consider doing in the hot zone won't feel good from higher levels. Just reach for that higher zone. Give others' the benefit of the doubt. Just like you do in every moment, they do the best they can. Their best may be awful, but that is because of where their emotions and beliefs were in that moment.

The meta-analysis published by Harvard in 2012[120] stated emphatically, "The absence of negative emotion is not the same as the presence of positive emotion." While evidence of this had been gradually accumulating, the meta-analysis evaluated 200 independent studies and reached this conclusion. This is a paradigm shift of monumental proportions.

If you have ever asked yourself why suffering in the world seems to be increasing, consider the definition of wellbeing (0 or above) to where true wellbeing occurs (+8 or above). This is not just something for insurance companies and the mental health profession to take note of. For implementation to help the masses, everyone has to adopt a new perspective about wellbeing. To truly prevent illness and obtain optimum health, we need to achieve sustainable emotional stances at + 8 or above.

Stoicism has a pervasive negative affect on society. Stoicism favors self-control and fortitude as the proper response to negative emotion. Culturally, we revere those individuals who are stoic in the face of tragedy. The Stoics were accurate in that negative emotions have a destructive effect on our mental processes, but their solution results in suppression of emotions, which contributes substantially to many societal problems.

In most modern situations, the Right Response to negative emotion is an adjustment of the perception, not fight or flight. True self-mastery requires learning how to interpret the messages and respond appropriately.

If we learn this technique and teach it to our employees and children, the world of the near future can exceed our highest dreams of a better world. Can you imagine less disease? Can you imagine a world where most people remain healthy and vital until old age? Can you imagine peace? Can you imagine how the world could be if the resources currently applied to hostilities were refocused toward increasing human thriving?

The difference between an intellectual understanding that perspective affects how we experience life and deliberately shifting our perspectives to make ourselves feel better is exhilarating. The first time I drove a car by myself I a very high feeling of elation even though I was just going to the post office. The first time we deliberately adjust a thought that feels bad to one that feels better creates the same type of empowered feeling.

We don't have to wait for others to do what we want before we can feel better. We can feel better now. It is a heady feeling, freeing and empowering. Our level of fear decreases substantially. We realize how bound up we have been by fear that others won't do what we "needed" them to do for us to feel better, and how bound up we have been that others might do things that would make us feel worse.

The science showing that the health benefits occur at + 8 and above should do a great deal to shift the current stoic attitudes that seem to reflect an attitude that if we're not prostrate with negative emotion, we're okay. Today it is very common for people to spend ten minutes sharing what is wrong in their life, their anger at this, their frustration at that, their

Chapter 16: Chronic Stress

grief about something else, and their irritation about something else before responding "I'm okay" when help is offered.

Yes, they are okay in that they are not in eminent danger of death from frustration, irritation, or even anger, but they are far from being the best they can be. This stems, I believe, somewhat from the belief that wellness is a cliff—it isn't.

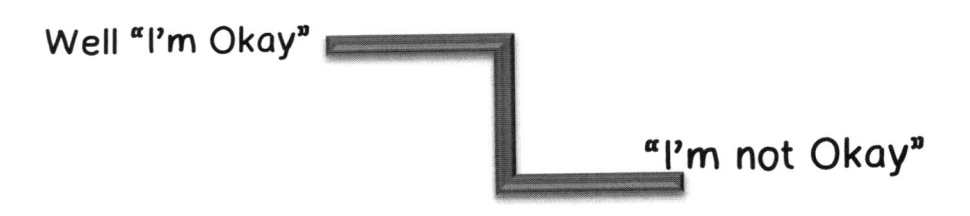

Well "I'm Okay"

"I'm not Okay"

Like so many other aspects of human thriving, it is a continuum. It is not a matter of being okay or not okay, it is a matter of how much less than optimal an individual is willing to tolerate.

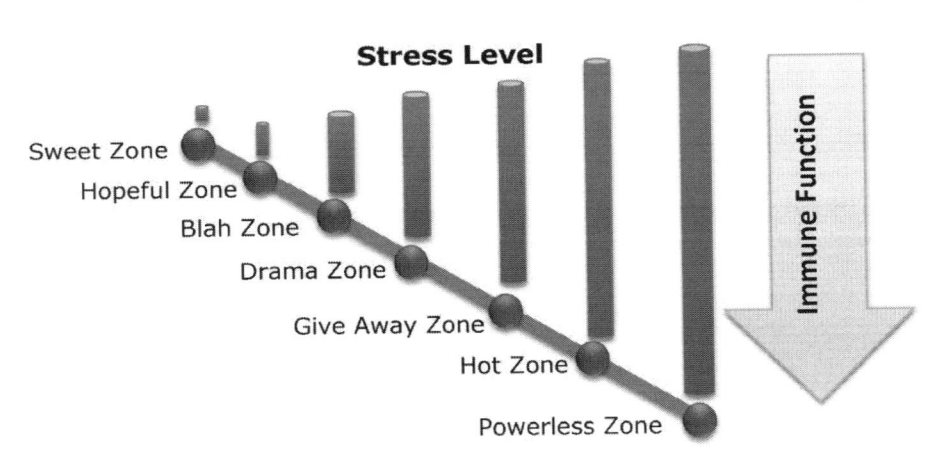

Stress Level

- Sweet Zone
- Hopeful Zone
- Blah Zone
- Drama Zone
- Give Away Zone
- Hot Zone
- Powerless Zone

Immune Function ↓

There is also the perception that needing help indicates weakness of some sort. While illness may make us physically weak and less mentally resilient, it does not mean we do not have the potential to be better. We know that many false premises have been passed down through the ages—false premises that hamper our ability to thrive. Obtaining help to move past a false premise is probably the only way to do so. Our beliefs, even when scientifically unsound, will be repeatedly proven to us via the filtering affect that decides what information reaches our conscious awareness.

Together, we can help one another thrive more. Individually, we can study and learn and make subtle shifts in our own minds that lead to increased thriving. Help does not mean baring our souls to a therapist. Help means accepting the help that is all around us. There is probably more help rejected because the person is "managing her suffering at a level where she can still function" than is actually received.

Accepting help does not mean we are weak. I've learned it takes strength to accept help. Rejecting help is often a sign of fear—fear that if I rely on someone else I may not be strong enough to face what comes in the future—fear that help may not always be there. But when one develops strong mental resilience, or a harty personality as it is sometimes labeled, the ability to navigate any adversity ahead is increased—not diminished.

Once an individual understands the relationship between emotional stance and behavior she is able to perceive much more about others' emotional states than those around her realize they are giving away. The secrets we think are so well-hidden from others are not obscured from those who understand this relationship. They may not understand every nuance, but they will have a far deeper understanding than those who do not see the relationship. Often, they understand more than the person they are observing about why he is reacting as he is.

As I said earlier, emotional and physical well-being exist along a continuum. It is all interrelated. Root cause solutions require an understanding of the larger picture.

Science has tended to study various aspects of humanity in isolation (Psychology, biochemistry, medical, neurological, consciousness, behavioral, sociology, criminology, genetics, etc.) These areas of science are often subdivided into specialties, such as addiction, immunology, cardiovascular disease, beliefs, epigenetics, and more.

Thoughts create the emotional feedback. The emotional stance affects body chemistry, bodily processes, behavior/actions, and ultimate outcomes. Circumstances do not create the emotion. Some individuals live in far less advantageous circumstances and are happy with their lives and receive the benefits of positivity.

Research into disparate outcomes evaluating situations with homogenous incomes vs. ones with more variety also reflects that it is not circumstances, but perception thereof, that matters.

Chapter 16: Chronic Stress

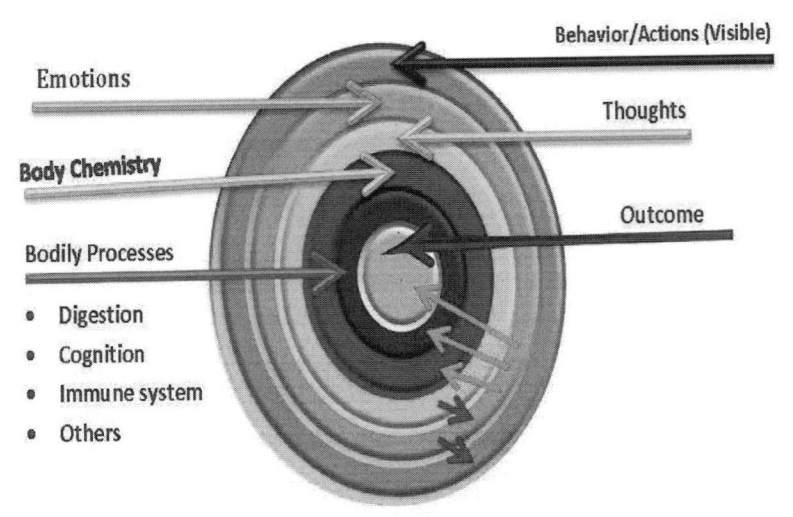

Behavior/Actions (Visible)
Emotions
Thoughts
Body Chemistry
Outcome
Bodily Processes
- Digestion
- Cognition
- Immune system
- Others

This chart indicates how the inner and outer world connect. Beginning with thoughts and traveling outward, the emotional response is followed by the behavior. Traveling inward from thoughts, the body chemistry changes, which effects bodily processes including digestion, cognition, and immune function. Those changes affect the outcome.

Consistent use of emotional guidance enables individuals to manage their emotional stance to higher levels on the EGSc. Stress decreases as higher levels on the EGSc are sustained.

Chronic, unmanaged stress will cause the harm, but the level of stress is a direct function of the mindset of the individuals involved.

It is the reason one individual can function well under stress and another falls apart. When the problem is healed at the root, or prevented at the root, true prevention occurs. Address the problem on any other level and adverse side effects often occur.

Mindset and Emergencies

To illustrate that mindset changes actions and that beneficial mindset adjustments can be made in an emergency, let's imagine such a situation. We are driving down a rural road and happen upon an accident scene that has clearly just occurred. There is an adult, unconscious, in the front seat and a child screaming in a car seat in the back seat. The engine is smoking. We are alone.

Most of us are conditioned to call 911 for help, which is a good practice. But from there, our mental process may make the difference between life and death for the occupants of the vehicle. From television, we may know the smoke from the engine could result in an explosion. Someone with a very negative mindset may believe she cannot rescue the people before the car blows up. Someone with a positive mindset may think he is lucky to be there so quickly, while there is still time to make a difference.

The belief will determine the action. The person who believes there is no time before the car blows up may not even attempt to help the child. Perhaps this person also has a physical malady that would hamper the effort. The point is not to judge the person's decision. The point is to demonstrate how the thinking process affects what action is taken, or not taken.

The person who believes he can rescue the occupants will go into action immediately. His body will cooperate with his decision—sending adrenaline that speeds up his physical actions and heightens his senses. If the occupants are strangers, he will probably rescue the child first. Mental processes may feel hypervigilant during the time the rescue is physically taking place—seeming almost dreamlike afterwards.

The temporary state of hypervigilance can provide additional benefits. For example, if the seatbelt of the unconscious adult were jammed, his mind might flash a picture of the beer bottle on the side of the road by the car in his mind, providing the quickest method of cutting the seatbelt.

This car accident scenario is dramatized to point out the effect of the underlying thoughts on the action taken. Modern societies teach us to take action—that action is the solution. While action is usually needed, addressing the mental state first results in better actions.

Let's return to the car accident scene. The person who happens on the scene this time is motivated more by guilt than by what he believes is possible. When he sees the child and the unconscious adult, he knows he must act because he would be unable to live with the guilt if he does not at least try. This person will die trying, if necessary. Not because he wants to die, but because he fears what life would be like for himself if he does not try. Guilt is a powerful motivator.

Although guilt is the primary motivator, this person's thoughts still fall on one side or the other of the belief that he can successfully rescue the people or he cannot successfully rescue them and will die in the attempt. Can you feel how, as he moves forward with a belief that he is going to die in this required (by guilt) effort, the belief/thoughts slow both his physical and mental processes? If you imagine the scene, instead of just reading the words on the page, you can feel how heavy those thoughts feel—sluggish is the word that comes to my mind.

On the flip side, the guilt-motivated individual who believes that he can successfully achieve the rescue will be aided by the hypervigilance mentioned above. In this individual, the guilt that drives the action may be hidden because they believe they can achieve the goal—his thoughts are not focused on how difficult life would be if he does not try. He may even imagine that this action will atone (in his own mind) for some regretted action from the past.

The motivation does not matter nearly as much as the perspective the individual takes about whether or not she will succeed.

Most of us have been trained to fall on one side of the other of the "I can do it" belief. Today, a growing number of individuals are consciously changing their default programming to a more positively focused perspective.

Let's take someone who is in the midst of deliberately transitioning a somewhat negative focus to a more positively focused one. He is not on the first day of this journey, but the more positively focused default is not automatic. As he sees the accident, the first thought may be that he is helpless, or that all he can do is call 911. But because he has been working toward changing negative default thinking, he feels the negative emotion accompanying the limiting thoughts, which triggers a conscious awareness that *he can change how he feels about this moment, in this moment.*

He tries a new thought, "I could at least get the child out of the car." This thought triggers different action—instead of waiting for rescue workers to arrive, he rushes to the car and frees the child. Depending on his thoughts while he performed that action, he may or may not also attempt to rescue the unconscious adult.

Do you see how the conscious decision to adjust ones thoughts changed the action taken? Can you also see how the level of stress experienced by the individual varied based on the mindset he held about his ability to help and his potential for success?

Chapter 17: Processes (How to Think Positive)

Today, you have the opportunity to transcend from a disempowered mindset of existence to an empowered reality of purpose-driven living. Today is a new day that has been handed to you for shaping. You have the tools, now get out there and create a masterpiece.

Steve Maraboli

In some of my programs, I teach more than 50 separate processes as tools my students can use to change their perceptions and reduce stress. Some processes provide immediate relief from negative emotions. Others assist students in reprogramming their neural pathways using beliefs the students have decided will serve their highest good. Some of the processes have little long-term effect; others have profound long-term effects.

The following pages outline processes that are effective methods of managing stress. One important aspect not usually considered by most teachers is that the specific process that will be most effective varies due to the current emotional state. There are other variables, but this one always matters.

In an earlier chapter, I mentioned that many commonly recommended happiness increasing/stress reducing techniques can be counter-productive. That's why, in the description for each process, I indicate what emotional state(s) the exercise is most suitable for. By now, you probably realize that in many cases the mental attitude is what determines whether it is productive or counter-productive.

Practical processes that help individuals navigate many of life's situations are scattered throughout TRUE Prevention. Examples provided in earlier chapters can provide insight and perhaps even epiphanies about behaviors that are not serving your highest good.

The purpose of the processes is to help you move up the EGSc and achieve the health, well-being, relationship, and success benefits that naturally occur when we are in higher zones. The EGSc is provided again below to make referencing it while you do the processes easier.

Emotional Guidance Scale (EGSc)

Sweet Zone
- Joy
- Empowered
- Passion
- Happy
- Inspired
- Optimism
- Fulfilled
- Appreciation
- Love
- Enthusiasm
- Positive Expectation
- Trust
- Serenity
- Freedom
- Awe
- Eagerness
- Belief
- Faith
- Satisfaction

Hopeful Zone
- Hopefulness
- Gratitude

Blah Zone
- Contentment
- Apathy
- Boredom
- Pessimism

Drama Zone
- Frustration
- Overwhelmed
- Irritation
- Disappointment
- Impatience

Give Away Zone
- Doubt
- Guilt
- Worry
- Discouragement
- Blame

Hot (Red) Zone
- Anger
- Revenge

Powerless Zone
- Hatred
- Insecurity
- Grief
- Powerlessness
- Hopelessness
- Rage
- Fear
- Depression
- Learned Helplessness
- Jealousy
- Unworthiness
- Despair
- Guardedness

↑ More Empowered Emotions

Immune system function

↓ Less Empowered Emotions

Follow Your Guidance

If you learn how to follow your EGS, you can reach sustainable happiness without learning any other processes. The other processes are tools that can assist you in finding the better-feeling perspectives your guidance is leading you to, but they are not necessary if you simply learn to understand and follow your guidance.

1. The first step is awareness that we have guidance.
2. The second is setting an intention to hear its messages.
3. The third is listening to the messages—they are often subtle.

In the beginning, we may only recognize that we received guidance in hindsight after we did not act upon it. The key here is not to beat ourselves up for failing to recognize it—that does not serve anyone. Recognizing we had guidance and did not heed it is a gift. It allows us to remember how it felt when we became aware of the guidance we overlooked, giving us a greater ability to realize the next time that those subtle messages are guidance.

Emotional guidance works just like the child's game, "Hot or Cold." While it does feel different to move from despair to anger than from anger to frustration, or from hope to passion, each of these steps is a step in the right direction; each is "getting warmer." The common aspect is that a feeling of relief (a releasing of tension or stress) is felt in each of these steps. The emotion that is in the "warmer" direction always feels better than emotions that are "getting colder."

Emotions are responses to thoughts. Thinking about something pleasing (past, present, or future) will create "getting warmer" emotional guidance. Thinking about something unpleasant (past, present, or future) will create "getting colder" emotional guidance. Everyone has the ability to make the choice to think about someone or something and focus on an aspect that feels good or an aspect that feels bad. The emotional guidance system provides feedback to each thought.

Emotional guidance leads to better feeling emotions, whether it is away from fear in a harmful environment or toward becoming the most we can imagine being. [121]

For many the hardest part of learning to follow the emotional guidance system is overcoming the conflicting instructions they received throughout life to use the opinions, expectations, and desires of others as guidance. The personal guidance provided by the emotional sensory system includes our goals in the order of importance the individual has assigned to them. On the surface it sounds very selfish, but an individual whose goals include being loving or respectful to others will be guided in a way that takes those goals into consideration.

The rational mind is not just filtered by beliefs. Expectations, emotional stance, and focus have a tremendous impact. That is one reason it is so hard for someone who has been in a chronic unhappy state to move to a better-feeling state using the rational mind. Habits of thought, like other habits, take time to change. Using the EGS as a guide to better-feeling thoughts, the rational mind is able to be reconditioned to support better-feeling emotional stances.

Our upbringing can have a significant effect on our ability to feel what emotion we are feeling. Some people were trained from young ages that being emotional was bad behavior. In many cases, emotions have been suppressed and these individuals may have a more difficult time labeling their emotions. However, the feeling of relief when a better-feeling thought is felt. Reaching for a feeling of relief will enable an individual with difficulty figuring out which zone he is in on the EGSc to use his guidance.

Both affirmations and setting intentions can help the individual who has subdued emotions to become more aware of them. Even individuals who have not been conditioned to suppress their emotions become more aware of subtle differences as they gain experience using the EGS.

First, it is critical to allow yourself permission to feel whatever you feel. If you feel guilty about how you feel, guilt is low on the EGS. You can't move to great feeling zones if you feel guilty. You feel what you feel. What you feel is valid, FROM YOUR CURRENT PERSPECTIVE. From your current perspective, what you feel is the appropriate response. From your current perspective, what you can feel. You cannot change how you feel about the situation without changing your perspective. Doing so will make you sick.

> When you find yourself feeling negative emotion about somebody else, recognize it as a situation where a Right Response would serve you well.

Your current perspective is valid and right from how you are perceiving the situation. That does not mean it is the only valid perspective about the topic. It does not mean it is the only perspective you can have bout the topic. It certainly does not mean it is the perspective that is best for your health, relationships, career, or overall well-being. In fact, if you feel anything less than excited expectation or joy or love or appreciation, there is a perspective that is more supportive of your highest good.

That being said, do not beat yourself up for not being in that perspective. The path to feeling better does not include self-criticism, or beating oneself about the head and shoulders with negativity. The path is one that supports you in becoming all you can become—which never requires condemnation of where you are—even if in your current perspective there are awful behaviors. It only requires recognition that you desire something better. Period.

Then, knowing you can move to better. You can't jump from awful to terrific in one fell swoop. It takes baby steps. But you know what, it does not take long between first baby steps and running. A baby step, followed by a baby step, followed by a baby step, with your EGS supporting you every step of the way, saying, "Yes, come this way. That's right. Good." Via emotional responses that feel better as you take those steps will help you build confidence. When you have confidence, you can begin moving faster. You begin trusting that changing perspective has rewards—sometimes great rewards. You begin accepting the new perspectives faster because you're no longer doubting the process. Once that happens you're off and running. You're still not leaping tall buildings—you're still going one step at a time, but the time between steps can be so short that on a single subject you can move from very disempowered to empowered in under an hour. Don't beat yourself up if you're not at this speed yet. If you have trouble with this, compare yourself to your prior self, comparing how it might have taken you months to move that as far as you now can in a day.

No one is at the same place on any subject. Comparing your results to another's is counterproductive. If you must compare yourself to another, compare your current self to your prior self. You will feel the positive reinforcement of progress forward.

Even if you forget for a while on a subject and wallow in negativity, you still know the process, at any time you can decide to begin the process on a sore subject. It is not about beating yourself up if you do not immediately apply the process to every area of your life.

You will also find that when you fix a problem in one area, it often helps in all other areas. A frustrating focus manifests in myriad ways throughout your day. It can include inept store clerks or waitresses, or inept driver's in front of you who fail to move when the light is green, it can involve teachers who seem to do things the hard way—whether it is letting you know the day before your child has to have something that you have to go to the store to buy or who mandate a field trip you have to take that conflicts with prior plans. It can include a manager at work who schedules you three weeks in advance on an important day you want off, but the policy does not allow you to request time-off more than two weeks in advance. It can involve someone putting the spaghetti back in the cupboard so when you pick it up, it all spills on the floor—the last box, now spread all over the floor instead of in the boiling pot on the stovetop—ten minutes before company is due to arrive.

When you move to a less frustrating zone, your brain will let you know the spaghetti is not in the cupboard correctly before it spills, you'll feel instincts to change lanes and not be behind the frustrating driver, you'll have a casual conversation with your manager where you mention the important date and they take note or tell you to go ahead and put in more than two weeks in advance. When you begin doing this deliberate work it almost feels magical.

Remember, the filters in our brain are designed as if we understand how they work. They literally hide information that is inconsistent with how they are set—whether it is in our best interest or not. They are not malicious or vindictive or determining our deservability (worthiness)—we do that. The filters only carry out their programming. Conscious programming is of enormous value.

The EGS provides reliable guidance and is appropriate for all emotional states.

Shift Your Focus

One of the most critical skills someone who is new to using his emotional guidance can develop is being able to deliberately change focus. It is the quickest path for relief in a distressing moment. Numerous techniques effectively help people change focus. In fact, most of the commonly taught techniques create a change of focus—that is why they work[5].

Changing focus is appropriate for emotional zones on the EGSc below Hopeful. A change of focus creates a distraction from a stressful perspective about the current topic of thought. Changes of focus provide immediate relief from uncomfortable emotions. Unless repeated frequently and consistently, a change of focus does not shift the underlying mindset or emotional stance. For that reason, I recommend changes of focus for immediate relief, but used in combination with techniques that change perspective and/or reprogram your neural pathways to more supportive default settings.

Changing focus is the easiest to achieve. It is quickest and provides immediate emotional relief from high stress/low emotional states. Unless it becomes habitual, it is only an in-the-moment solution. Although changing focus can provide fast relief, if the topic that does not feel good is encountered frequently, doing the work to move up the EGSc on that topic is well worth the effort.

If an old topic that is just frequently in your mind because you keep remembering it, you may be better served by focusing your thought elsewhere as much as possible until you have more experience at this. If a topic with a distressing or less than optimal emotional stance associated with it is one that you encounter often, working your way up the EGSc is the preferred long-term solution.

As you learn, it is very helpful to remember that you have neurological pathways that will take you back to old thoughts and old ways of thinking. This is temporary if you persist in focusing on the new way(s) of thinking your neural pathways will change. I believe this is the reason many people feel their low emotional state is hopeless. If they do not understand that

---

[5] Helping others, exercise, being in nature, listening to music, etc. are all methods of shifting focus.

finding themselves back in the old emotional place is a normal part of the growth process that will subside over time, it is easy to give up.

Repetitive thoughts, whether assigned a label (such as OCD) or not, are simply the result of a neural pathway that is easier to travel due to repetitive use. New paths can be created.

If you lived in a house near the woods and took a walk each morning, initially you would probably travel the path with the least amount of brush and branches to move, etc. Perhaps you would follow a deer trail. After a while, walking that path every day would create a larger path, even easier to walk. If you decided for some reason that you wanted to walk a different route it would be more difficult, you would have branches to move, perhaps logs to walk over, possibly thorns protruding into the path, etc. You can do it, but it is easier to walk the existing worn path. Also, sometimes, when you were not consciously focused on taking the new path you would automatically revert to the old path, discovering yourself walking down the old path. Or perhaps you have moved and found yourself, after a long day at work, automatically heading to your former home. Eventually your circuits all line up and even when you are on auto-pilot, you drive to your current residence.

The biggest key is not to be upset when you find your thoughts on the old path. Just recognize where you are and move to where you want to be. Criticizing yourself for being on the old path is counter-productive. When we decide a thought path no longer serves us we have to clear a little brush to walk another path but it is worth the effort and it is only difficult at first. The second time is easier than the first and by the 10th, you cannot even recall how difficult it was the first time.

You cannot STOP thinking about something by trying to stop thinking about it because when you try to stop thinking about the thing you don't want to think about, you are thinking about it.

You can, however, decide to think about something else and every time you begin thinking about the topic you don't want to think about have something more pleasant to think about already planned as diversions.

At first, you will still have the unwanted thoughts a bit but you will spend less time with them and more time on the more pleasant thoughts.

KNOW that you can change your thoughts, even habitual thoughts. You have control. *You think them; they do not think you.* I would not label repetitive thoughts with a label that gives them more power than they deserve. With consistent effort, everyone can change their thought paths. The more power given to labels, the harder it is to believe in your ability to change and to find the hope that you can do it.

One reason developing skills in changing focus is critical is that it is the only type of process a new student can use to change a painful emotional state quickly. For someone who is considering self-harm, the ability to change focus quickly can be lifesaving. At low emotional states, finding a better

feeling thought can seem impossible if you have not been taught skills to help you. It can feel as if you'll never feel better. The Focus Shift process empowers you with a way to shift your focus to a better feeling thought when you need it the most.

I recommend this process for everyone. It is best prepared for when you are in the Hopeful or Sweet Zone, but the process is actually used when you are emotionally below the Hopeful Zone. This process is one of the few that provide quick relief when you are in the Powerless Zone.

Focus Shift—The List

When you are in a good mood, make a list of simple things that make you feel good when you think about them. The list should be things you can actually enjoy—not something you want (like winning the lottery). My list has things like sunrises, sunsets, flowers, babies, little red haired girls, doing something for someone else, and remembering overcoming obstacles in the past. On my list, I also have ice cream to remind myself of a specific time when I felt cared for. There is no right or wrong as long as it is something that makes you feel good when you think about it.

Keep your list in your wallet or purse. If you ever find yourself in an emotional state where you can't think of anything that feels better, all you have to do is remember you have the list. Take it out and look at it.

One time, many years ago, I was in that low place where I was unable to think a single good feeling thought. Remembering the list, but not anything that was on it, I found it in my purse. Reviewing it, there were no babies in the vicinity. It was midafternoon so no sunrises or sunsets were out. Then I saw flowers on the list. It was January, so even my yard lacked flowers. Then I remembered the grocery store has flowers.

I got in the car, drove to the grocery store, and spent about half an hour in the floral section. I admired the flowers, smelled the flowers, enjoyed the pretty colors, and the floral scents. By the time I left the store, my mood was greatly improved. I never again returned to such a low mood, because when my emotional state begins to decline, I take action sooner.

The list must be made when you feel good because that is when you can remember thoughts and memories that feel good to you.

My trip to the grocery store did not change any of the facts of the situation that had caused the low mood in the first place, but by shifting to a higher mood my mind was able to see the situation in a better light. Solutions that were not mentally accessible from the lower emotional state occurred to me.

In the lowest emotional states, changing ones focus is the quickest path to feeling better in the moment. When the mood is that low, the most critical thing anyone can do is find a way to feel better. Sometimes that means sleeping.

Focus is the easiest aspect of our emotional stance to change quickly. Changing beliefs that do not serve us provides more progress, but changing a belief that is at the root of a low emotional state is very difficult when one is at a low emotional state. It is better to work on changing unsupportive beliefs when feeling hopeful or better.

A change of focus is a powerful tool. It is an easy one to practice and can be done under any circumstances.

Deliberately Choose Happy Thoughts

These processes are very simple and are recommended for any emotional state below the Sweet Zone. When you're in the Sweet Zone, real life feels better than the process.

Basically, all you have to do is make a decision to deliberately focus on something that feels better. It can be something pleasing from your past, present, or future that creates a "getting warmer" feeling. With practice, the ability to focus oneself into a good feeling state regardless of circumstances can be developed.

Numerous enhancements can be used to give this process more power.

For example, I plan my life so that I always have something to look forward to. Then I intentionally give attention to the anticipated event and savor it now. I love to travel, so it is rare that I do not have a vacation to look forward to enjoying, but I can also enjoy vacations from my past by remembering the best parts of them.

I've learned that planning a vacation further in advance increases my enjoyment of it. I savor the anticipation of it and then enjoy the actual trip. When I have a short planning horizon, the amount of enjoyment I receive from the trip is less.

It does not have to be a vacation. It can be anticipating a holiday with family, a meal at a special restaurant, finishing a class or an education, reading a good book, an upcoming movie release, the meal on your plate in front of you, a bottle of your favorite wine chilling in the refrigerator, a warm fire in the fireplace, a comfortable chair, a good friend, the feel of your body when you stretch, and more.

How many times have you eaten a good meal while thinking about something that diminished the experience?

This process is about being aware and deliberately choosing thoughts that feel good. The intention is what makes it a process. Most people simply allow whatever is top of their mind or in front of them to have their attention. We can do better than that—we can choose the object of our attention based on how it feels when we think about it.

Positive Affirmations

Positive Affirmations are recommended for the current emotional stance reaching for no more than one zone higher than the current emotional stance. Basically, you can do affirmations from any emotional stance as long as the affirmation is believable from your current position. Positive affirmations are one of the most widely taught techniques and they probably cause the most harm. They cause harm, not because the process is bad or defective, but because most teachers do not differentiate between when Positive Affirmations are beneficial and when they are inappropriate or counterproductive.

Positive affirmations have been scientifically shown to be counterproductive when the individual does not believe the affirmation. The person can say the positive affirmation, but internally the mind refutes it, which makes the underlying belief stronger. Positive affirmations should only be used when they do not create this mental backlash. In other words, make adjustments that are not huge stretches from the existing belief on the specific topic. For example, affirming you love your job when you hate it just reinforces the aspects of the job you do not enjoy.

The key to using Positive Affirmations is to lean in direction of the desired emotion. This approach, applied consistently over time, results in amazing and delightful changes. If your emotional stance is in the Drama Zone, reach for another emotion in the same zone that feels slightly better or for one in the Blah Zone. If you attempt to affirm a thought that would be in the Hopeful Zone you're likely to have pushback in your own mind. Move to the Blah Zone and stabilize there by affirming thoughts you believe in the Blah Zone. Once you are stable, move to new thoughts that feel even better.

It is always the underlying mental attitude that determines whether something is counterproductive. For example, knowing that exercise makes one feel better is helpful when we actually exercise. When we feel bad and don't take the physical action of exercising, there is a tendency to add guilt for not exercising to the existing negative emotion—perhaps starting a downward spiral. When we understand how to adjust our perceptions to feel better, we can counter any guilt we begin to feel before it adds to our emotional burden.

Here is an example. The person is afraid of public speaking and shy about interacting with strangers.

Affirmation: I am a charismatic public speaker.

Internal dialogue: "Who are you trying to fool? You couldn't talk your way out of a paper bag. If you get up on the stage they'll laugh you right off."

Affirmation: I am a charismatic public speaker.

Internal dialogue: "Still trying to convince yourself of that? You can try forever; you don't have what it takes to be on stage."

Instead of leaping from the current belief (I am not even good at interpersonal communication. There is no way I can speak on stage in front of hundreds of people.) all the way to the desired belief take a baby step.

Affirmation: Today I will speak to a stranger, even if I am afraid. The worse that can happen is I'll look foolish.

Internal dialogue: "There is someone. Oh, this is scary."

Action: Walking toward stranger.

Internal dialogue: "Just say hello. Or ask him what time it is."

Internal dialogue: "I can do this."

Action: "Hi, isn't it a pretty day?"

Internal dialogue: "Wow. I got that out without tripping over my tongue. I can do this. What should I do next?"

Internal dialogue: "Tomorrow I'll speak to two strangers."

Positive affirmations that reach too far cement undesired beliefs more firmly in our minds. Remember, it is possible to feel hopeful that you will actually be able to have two conversations with strangers tomorrow and frightened about the idea of being on stage talking to a room full of strangers.

Pay attention to the internal dialogue. If your inner critic is responding, you have two choices. The easiest is to take a smaller step that your critic won't attack. The longer term solution is to kill your inner critic.

Unlike most processes, the emotional zone this one works in depends on using it correctly (taking small steps toward better feeling thoughts) rather than the emotional stance the individual is in. That being said, in the lowest emotional states it can be difficult to find a better-feeling thought so other processes will be effective faster, especially in the Powerless Zone.

Think Positive

I include this as a process to attempt to provide some clarification and perhaps some emotional relief. "Be positive," "Stay positive," "Keep your chin up," and "Don't let it get you down" are all forms of advice given frequently, without answering the question of how to actually achieve it.

First, if you've heard this advice and been unable to follow it—the reason is that without instructions, it is meaningless advice.

In a study of cancer patients and nurses about the definition of "being positive," it was defined "as maintaining some sort of normality without letting cancer have a detrimental effect on daily living." Nurses identified hope, acceptance, fighting spirit and looking on the bright side as definitions of 'being positive.' Nurses and patients identified environment and support of family, friends, and health professionals as factors that influence patient attitudes. Patients also identified other peoples' attitudes as important. It was concluded that "Being positive" must be acknowledged as central to being able to cope with cancer and its treatment. The ability of nurses to care for patients with cancer and help them to remain positive will be improved if they develop a better understanding of the meaning of "being positive" for patients, and how other peoples' attitudes affect their state of mind.[122]

> *Someone who puts a smiling face forward who is screaming, or deathly afraid, on the inside is not in a positive frame of mind and the contradiction between their outward face and inward feelings is actually detrimental to their recovery and well-being.*

This definition does not go nearly far enough and it may be one reason research into the benefit of positivity on health has not shown consistent results.

What does a beneficial positive focus look like? First, we have to look inside the mind to the thoughts. The outer face can be more or less positive but authenticity is another element that is beneficial to health so I highly recommend consistency between the inner and outer mood. If you do not want people around you while you feel awful, retreat, but only if you are doing positive work on moving forward. Sometimes, from the worse perspectives, this is the best way. But do not retreat for long and if you are not making progress, ask for help from someone who understands how to change perspectives to ones that are more positive.

The mind of the positively focused person has a belief that things can get better. The best way to cultivate this belief is to practice using one's emotional guidance and develop confidence in the process. Then apply processes appropriate to the current mood to shift perspective to a more positively focused one.

It also involves being less judgmental, angry, unforgiving, and just plan unloving toward others—whether strangers, family, friends, or enemies. When you judge another as lacking, your guidance is telling you there is a better perspective you can find about the person/situation. The negative emotion you feel is not telling you that the person/situation is awful—it is telling you that the perspective you are taking about the situation is not serving your highest good. The same is true when you are angry with someone else. When you refuse to forgive, you harm yourself, not the other person.

The perspective that your anger toward another punishes them is in error. It is possible for someone to feel anger toward me and I can be completely oblivious toward his or her feelings. Or, I can choose to think they are just living in the hot zone and they are the only one who can change that, the emotional zone they chose to live in—consciously or unconsciously—has nothing to do with me.

The perspective that refusing to forgive another punishes them in some way is also in error. Yes, it can be a catalyst for emotional pain—if they decide your forgiveness is important and necessary to their well-being. But whether or not to take that perspective is completely up to them—you do not have a say. I know people who are angry and unforgiving toward people who are no longer alive. If you are one of those people, imagine how it would feel if you weren't habitually angry. Imagine it, and feel it, and move toward that feeling. If you know someone who is habitually angry, the best thing you can do for them is to imagine them happy and to focus on your own happiness. It's contagious.

Setting Intentions

Setting intentions is a form of goal setting. When you set intentions to do certain things, it sensitizes the filters that decide which information will be sent to your conscious mind, highlighting information in alignment with your intentions.

I used to work with a very quick-witted COO from New York who frequently responded while I was still formulating my response in our executive meetings. Often, this took the conversation in a new direction and my opportunity to add value passed without my input. I began setting the intention "The best answers I can think of will come to me quickly" as I walked to the boardroom for our meetings. My responses became faster. The COO was no longer always ahead of me in his responses. I still remember his face the first time I answered ahead of him.

Intentions can be set for one's life—much like a mission statement. They can be set for a year, a month, a day, a relationship, a journey, a conversation. Setting intentions is a very versatile form of goal setting.

Intentions can be general or specific. You can set a goal that your decisions will always lean toward your highest good. You can set an intention to be aware of situations where you can be of benefit to others.

What would you like to have more of in your life? What would you like to do better in your life?

I like goal setting. I had a 1, 2, 5, and 20-year plan when I was 21. I am convinced that many of my successes were the result of setting specific goals.

I like setting intentions because they do not require a lot of preparation or thought. They help one be in the flow more often when the intention is to be the best you can in the moment.

Setting intentions is good for any level on the EGSc. Much like with the Positive Affirmation process, the key is to set intentions you believe you can achieve. The difference between Setting Intentions and Positive Affirmations is that Setting Intentions is about something you are going to do and the outcome you desire from the activity.

Do you have an area of your life where you often feel just a little less than you want to be? Try setting an intention for what you would like better and see what happens.

Forgiving

Many people refuse to forgive someone who has hurt them not realizing that harboring ill will toward another harms their health, their enjoyment of life, and their potential for success.

Refusing to forgive is like walking through life with a leg shackle attached to one's leg—it weighs you down, slows you down, and holds you back.

You've learned a lot about the connection between emotional state and behavior. Our best possible behavior when we are in the Powerless Zone is far less than the best behavior we offer when we are in the Sweet Zone. The other thing is that none of us wake-up in the morning and decide to do less than the best we are able to do that day. Even when our behavior is far less than our best possible, or best ever, we are doing the best we can in the current emotional state.

Between knowing that forgiveness is the best choice for my personal well-being (and the best choice for your well-being as well) and that whatever happened, it was the best the person could do in that moment makes it easier to forgive. Research is indicating that forgiveness is powerful medicine for the one who forgives[123].

Another way to reach for forgiveness is attempting to see the situation from their point of view. This can be an especially beneficial method when the unforgiven party has apologized[124] or if you are aware of a history that might have made the person more likely to do what they did.

The other piece is what I call unbundling. In many instances, we bundle forgiveness with allowing someone back into our lives. But the two things are not the same and can be unbundled. It is possible to forgive someone for something and make a decision not to have that person in your life. They are separate decisions and you get to decide how you want to handle any situation in your life.

It is also possible to love someone but choose not to have that person in your life. Loving and being involved do not have to be bundled. Many times the reason an individual does not want to forgive is because they do not want to risk a repeat of the event that felt so bad to them. By unbundling forgiveness from resuming a relationship, forgiveness may come more easily to you.

I recommend unbundled forgiveness for anyone who is holding onto hurt or anger, in any emotional stance.

Nature

A lot of research points to the happiness increasing benefits of being in nature. Being outside has a positive influence on mood. Spending time in nature is recommended as a way to temporarily reduce stress at every zone on the EGSc.

Time outside in nature on a daily basis can help a person deal with high levels of stress. Nature was one of my "go to" stress relieving activities before I understood my EGS.

Going out in nature has a positive effect on mood that may last longer than the actual time spent in nature. However, as in many other activities, what you think while you are in nature will have a tremendous impact on how beneficial the time in nature is. Being in nature is not a magic panacea that changes your perception. It can help change your perception, if your thought processes while you spend time outdoors support this. However, thought processes that move down the EGSc can be followed while in nature. I recommend care be taken to be consciously aware of the thought paths your mind wanders while you enjoy the great outdoors. If they are traveling a negative path, redirect them down a more productive path.

> Adjusting your thoughts toward better-feeling perspectives will provide the most benefit to you.

Time in nature is a temporary mood improvement tool that works when the mindset accompanying the time in nature is positive. The benefits may extend past the time spent in nature, but it does not create lasting changes unless the time is used to adjust ones mindset to more positive perspectives.

Exercise

Exercise is often recommended as a way to reduce stress, and if used correctly, it is effective. There is a lot of research supporting the benefits of exercise. I have not seen any research that compared a group who exercised as usual compared to a group that received stress management classes and exercised. I would like to see that research.

Exercise is a beneficial, stress-reducing practice. During one particularly stressful period of my life, I exercised eleven times each week. Exercise was my main stress-relieving outlet and it was very effective. But, exercise did nothing to shift my focus so I saw my thoughts from a better perspective. Combining the two would have made the situation less stressful.

One of the reasons I love the Make Play OK™ campaign is that it makes exercise fun instead of something likely to invoke guilt and add to the stress load.

I recommend exercise, but not as an isolated solution. At a minimum, ones EGS should be used in conjunction with exercise to help adjust thought patterns to less stressful perspectives.

Exercisers are cautioned:
- Not to be self-critical of their exercise achievements.
- Not to feel guilty if they miss a day;
- Not to dwell on things that bring up negative emotion while exercising (and other times).

Someone who has a habit of self-criticism who takes up an otherwise healthy exercise routine may use exercise as another reason to be self-critical. The negative emotion from the self-criticism sabotages their efforts and reduces their emotional stance.

See the Potential in Others and in Self

This is not the same as seeing the good in others. While that is a good practice, seeing the potential looks deeper. Seeing the good usually refers to seeing good that is manifesting in their experience. An example would be to see the kind heart of the failing student.

Seeing the potential in others, while not overlooking the kind heart of the aforementioned student, would also see within the student the potential to thrive in school instead of fail. I recommend this process for everyone to use to the best of their abilities.

Seeing the potential in others begins with an understanding that our best behavior in any moment is impacted by our emotional state in that moment. The current emotional state has significant impacts on all of the following:

Behavior	Intelligence	Emotional Intelligence
Health	Well-being	Resilience
Relationships	Motivation	Creativity

In addition, ES directly impact decisions including ones involving diet, exercise, alcohol, drugs, and risky behavior. Our society has a tendency to judge individuals based on their current behavior. I will continue with the example of the student who is failing.

When a student is failing, there is a tendency to assume she will not succeed in school; that in fact, she is not capable of being successful in school. If we look below the surface and find that this student is being abused at home or bullied at school, we will realize that she is lower on the EGSc than she could be. Understanding that, we can see that given a better situation and knowledge of how to move to higher levels on the EGSc, she might become a successful student.

This practice is important for both the person making the judgment and the student. For the person making the judgment, we spent some time in Chapter 4 explaining how our stress level rises and our emotional stance decreases when we judge another negatively.

For the student, in Chapter 13 I discussed mirror neurons and brain sync. Whoever has the more dominant belief about the student's potential for success will influence the other—without words having to be spoken.

> *Technology is nothing. What's important is that you have a faith in people, that they're basically good and smart, and if you give them tools, they'll do wonderful things with them.*
>
> **Steve Jobs**

In general, you can assume that someone behaving in undesirable ways has negative emotions that have not been responded to in of the three constructive methods. The best response to most negative emotion in modern society involves 'Right Responses[125] (RRs). This involves some action or a deliberate and conscious change in mindscape.

Emotions provide information to guide us. The other two appropriate responses are Fight (non-violent assertive resistance) or Flight. Suppressing or denying emotions is dysfunctional and leads to many other problems.

If we are judging an unhappy person based upon their behavior, we are not seeing their potential. When we see their potential, we are more likely to inspire them to achieve more of their potential. Potential is a terrible thing to waste.

If we judge ourselves based on our past actions without taking into consideration our emotional state when we made the choices we are judging, we significantly underestimate our potential.

> I know in my heart that man is good. That what is right will always eventually triumph. And there's purpose and worth to each and every life.
> **Ronald Reagan**

Developing a habit of seeing others for their potential, rather than who they are being in the moment, makes us inspiring to them. By seeing what they cannot see in themselves, we help show them the way to become more of the potential within them.

Humanity has been operating in a way that hinders its ability to thrive. Much like attempting to run a marathon with a weight strapped to one leg would hinder progress, misinterpretation of our EGS has been impairing our ability to thrive. We now know enough to unlock the chains that have been holding us back.

Use your intention setting skills to set an intention to see the potential in yourself and others. I encourage you to reinforce this on a daily basis. You will love who you become.

Meditation

On the stress scale in Chapter 8, meditation is above passion, indicating higher cognitive ability and lower stress. This is because meditation is a process that clears the mind of habitual thought, clearing the way for insight. Emotions respond to thought. Meditation provides a respite from thought and therefore from emotion. Meditation is the most researched of the recommended processes. The documented results indicate that meditation is life-enhancing in every area of life.

I recommend that each individual mediate fifteen minutes per day. I also recommend meditation as a tool to regain one's center if the day's events have taken them off-kilter.

I had the experience of many days throughout my career that were derailed by the day's events. Taking the time to meditate was the best alternative, by far, for both the employee and the employer.

Some people object to meditation because they believe it is a religious practice. It is true that meditation is part of the religious rituals of many belief systems. However, rejecting meditation on religious grounds is akin to a non-Catholic refusing to use candles because Catholics use candles in their religious rituals. It is the intent of your meditation, not the act itself, that makes meditation a religious practice or not.

The meditation I recommend for the daily practice is not based on a religious practice. It involves lightly focusing on something, it can be a candle, the sound of an air conditioner, the hum of an engine, your own breathing, or any other object of attention that is sufficient to focus upon that does not bring forth an emotional response. Choose a noise you find soothing.

Sit or lay quietly focusing on the object of your attention. Breathe deeply and slowly, pulling air fully into your lungs and then slowly releasing. If distracting thoughts show up, breathe them away by refocusing on the object you have chosen to focus on. If you feel tense, you can offer yourself suggestions such as "I am feeling more relaxed" but such suggestions are optional. And, do not use a suggestion that you are attempting to force yourself to believe (see Positive Affirmations).

If you want the practice to be more religious, you can ask your deity to help you gain the maximum benefit from the practice before you begin.

The second meditation practice that is highly beneficial to individuals who practice it is mindfulness. At its essence, mindfulness means staying in the now—not thinking about past or future. Simply focusing on what is happening right now. I have seen mindfulness used with significant success in a number of circumstances, including disabling PTSD. There are a number of good books on the topic and classes are available in most areas.

While I recommend mindfulness to some of my students, I do not recommend it globally. Personally, I like savoring the past and future. For someone who is able to focus on the positives of the past, present, and future without dwelling on the negatives, I do not recommend it. I tell them they can try mindfulness, but savoring is an emotion high on the EGS that is beneficial to ones wellbeing. On the other hand, for individuals with a tendency to catastrophize or ruminate (dwell) on the negatives of the past, present, or future, incorporating mindfulness[126] while they adjust their underlying beliefs can be highly beneficial.

A third type of meditation I highly recommend is Open Heart Meditation. I recommend this type to anyone who is drawn to it. Open Heart meditation helps us connect more fully with those with whom we share the planet. I am working on a guided Open Heart Meditation CD. The daily meditation I recommend to everyone brings me to a state of peaceful relaxation. Open Heart Meditation brings me to a state where I feel love for everyone around the world. It is a highly positive emotional state.

I'd like to mention a fourth type of meditation. Transcendental Meditation (TM) has been heavily researched and the results of the practice demonstrate significant health and wellbeing benefits.

In some ways, meditation is a way to put the five loud senses on mute so we become more aware of the subtler perceptions available to us. The EGS will help each individual determine which practices will be most beneficial to them.

Go General

Anytime someone is in a low emotional state, he is focused on specifics. For example, if a health problem has him upset, he is focused on the specific aspect of his body that is not functioning the way he wants it to. As long as we are alive, more of our body is functioning well than not. He could have a kidney that is bad, but his mind, heart, lungs, arms, legs, eyes, nose, tongue, skin, and so much more are functioning perfectly. The narrow focus on the specific feels bad. As we deliberately think more generally, about our entire body, we feel better.

When you have some quiet time, play with the concept of going general to feel better. If you are upset about a situation at work, mentally take a step back and identify how specifically you are focused. Are you focused on something that happened for only a few minutes out of an entire week? Are you focused on something one person out of 100 did? Are you focused on one day out of an entire year? If you feel negative emotion about it, you are focused specifically.

This is true even if you are looking at something you perceive as a global problem. If you focus on world hunger, you can bring yourself to your knees with the hit of negative emotion. From that position, you cannot be effective in resolving the problem. In that negative state, your cognitive abilities are severely restricted.

If you step back and think about how many people have adequate food, your emotional stance will improve. You may immediately think again of those who do not—it is your habit of thought if this issue is on your mind frequently. Deliberately think again of those who have enough to eat. While you are in that higher emotional state, ask yourself, "How can more people have enough to eat?" Give time a chance to bring solutions. When you find yourself thinking about the problem, begin telling yourself things like, "We'll figure it out soon" or "We're making technological advances all the time, a solution could be found any time now" or "There are a lot of smart people in the world who would like to solve this problem.

I am not the only one who is concerned. The right idea will come to one of us."

Remember, it does not matter what the problem is, your ability to solve it is diminished when you feel negative emotion. That means the most you can do from that negative state is make yourself feel better. From that better-feeling state, you have more resources to help you find a solution.

This process is recommended for all zones below the Hopeful Zone. Increase your happiness first, then solve problems.

Let's try it now. Get a blank piece of paper. It can have lines or be completely blank. Write down something that has been bothering you. Then think about the issue by asking yourself questions, such as "What is the opposite of this?" and "What does the big picture look like?" as well as "Will this matter tomorrow (or in 5 years)?"

Put the issue that is bothering you in a broader context. Then feel how your emotion about the topic shifts.

If your emotions become worse, you are going more specific, not more general. Be patient with yourself and try again. If you have been practicing the negative thoughts for a long time it can be a little bit like starting the lawn mower the first time in the spring, which means it requires a little more effort to get going but once you start, it is easier the next time.

General to specific

When one's emotional stance is at the lower end of the EGSc, going more general will invoke better-feeling emotions. When you're on the high end of the EGSc, it is good to go more specific. You can actually bring yourself to a state akin to a natural high by going more specific while in the Sweet Zone. The key is to go as specific as you can while still feeling good.

Talking about doing it may seem difficult, but doing it is easy because your mind helps you when you are in the Sweet Zone. Before you begin this exercise, think about a topic where your emotional set point is in the Sweet Zone for a minute or two. This primes your mind to think of more thoughts in the Sweet Zone.

Before you go more specific with the topic you've chosen, I'm going to give you an example with something simple. The following is how I personally go more specific when I'm working and want to increase my cognitive abilities by increasing my emotional stance:

> I love sitting here feeling the morning sun on my skin. Soaking in the warmth feels so wonderful I appreciate the sun, rising every morning without any effort at all on my part. I love

the way the birds sing every morning, greeting the sun. I know the birds enjoy it too, that makes me feel more connected to nature and my world. Oh look, my hydrangeas are blooming! I love the big fluffy flowers. I always wanted big hydrangeas in my yard and now I have them. I am so blessed. Everything I ever dreamed of having is mine, and so much more than I ever imagined.

To be able to live and know that no matter what happens in life, I can find a perspective where I feel good is so amazing. I want everyone to have this freedom to live fully. Oh, look, the finches are on the birdfeeder. I love living where they come to feed. I love the big open area behind my house. I love watching the birds and the butterflies enjoy all the flowers I planted. I love how peaceful it is out here. My coffee tastes so good this morning.

:::stretching::: It feels so good to stretch. I love my body, its health, the way it helps me accomplish what I want to do and how wise it is. When I get a cut, it knows exactly what to do to heal. When I eat, my body knows how to take exactly what it needs and deliver it to the cells that need it. When I feel good, my body responds by feeling wonderful. It is awesome to live in such a smart body. I'm so glad I don't have to think about making sure my body does what it needs to in order to provide me with a wonderful home. It just knows what to do. I love that I can do things I've done many times, like riding a bicycle, driving a car, typing, or brushing my teeth and I don't have to think about the specifics. I just move into the motions and my body takes over. Isn't that wonderful? It is so much nicer than if I had to think about each little step in the process.

Life is so good and just becomes better all the time. Delightful little surprises, like the butterfly that is flitting around my flowers, show up to surprise and delight me.

I love our planet. It is so beautiful. I love the way the plants know what to do, just like my body knows what to do. They begin growing at just the right time. I could tell the month and almost the day by when my peonies bloom, when the first rose of the season blooms, when the Daffodils, hyacinth, tulips, pansies, and grape hyacinths bloom. It is all so coordinated and all I had to do was plant them. They are so reliable, coming back year after year. I love the resilience of nature, and how everything is interwoven. I love being outside and being able to begin my day this way. I love the way the rain comes and washes everything, the way the wind comes to dry it off, and how the rainbows appear when the sun shines while it is raining elsewhere. I love the absolute beauty of our planet, the stars in the sky at night and the way the moon seems so close as it lights up the night sky. I am so blessed to live on this magnificent planet with so much variety and beauty.

Can you feel how after writing out details of what you are appreciating you would feel very stable in the Sweet Zone? Do you feel the way it adds emphasis to things that I see every day, such as the flowers in my yard? By doing that, each time I see the flowers I am reminded of how good I can feel. By affirming the wisdom of my body[6] I increase my conscious trust in it. This reduces any concerns or worry I may have about a body declining because of age. By the way, research has shown that our expectations about aging are what we tend to experience. This exercise can be done verbally, orally, or simply in your head. Writing it is the most powerful when you are doing a general appreciation of life like I've done above.

Remember, this exercise is best done when you are in the Sweet Zone on the EGSc. It can be done in the Hopeful Zone. Below the Hopeful Zone it can be counterproductive.

It is a good exercise for increasing your stability in the Sweet Zone. Whether you rarely feel the emotions in the Sweet Zone or you live most of your life there, the stabilizing influence of this exercise will increase your time in the Sweet Zone.

If you are in the Sweet Zone, try this exercise now.

Appreciation (not gratitude)

Many teachers teach gratitude as a way of increasing positive emotions. I prefer to teach appreciation. For about one third of people, there is no real difference, but for two thirds, appreciation is the more powerful practice.

The reason for this differentiation has to be explained on the quantum level. Despite all Webster's attempts, each of us have our own meanings attached to words and situations. On the quantum level, the words have vibrations that reflect the definition the person has for the word.

I'll provide an example using the word peace. To me it means a feeling I have been able to find inside my own heart where I feel love for everyone on the planet. I have learned that by placing peace in my own heart, I can feel at peace with the world—even as a war rages somewhere on the planet.

---

[6] By expecting my body to be smart and know what to do, there is coherence on the quantum level that is of great benefit to me.

I am not intertwined with the war, I am entwined with peace on the quantum level.

For many others, "peace" currently means something longed for but unattainable. That meaning has an entirely different vibration to it than the one I mean when I say or think the word peace.

I teach appreciation instead of gratitude because most people perceive appreciation in the same way. It is a feeling that is closely related to love.

I find that people seem to define gratitude in three distinct ways:
1. I am so grateful that someone bigger/better/more powerful than I am did for me something I could not do for myself,
2. I have to find a way to pay X back for doing this wonderful thing for me, I am indebted to X for the help I received in my time of need, and
3. A feeling of appreciation

Appreciation is defined as: the recognition and enjoyment of the good qualities of someone or something.

If you compare #1 and #2 to the emotional stances on the EGSc, you will notice that they are very different degrees of empowerment from appreciation. Appreciation is a completely empowered feeling. The other two definitions are at a much lower emotional state. Sometimes seemingly slight differences can make a difference. For this reason, I teach appreciation but I do not teach gratitude.

In the long run, each of us is better served seeing ourselves as able to help ourselves but appreciative of help that comes to us.

There has been much research on the feeling of helplessness that clearly shows that those who feel helpless give up and do not even try. This is true of both animals and humans.

Some people will say you do owe someone who has helped you. I disagree. Here is why: I teach human thriving for a living. While I charge for my programs and books, as I move through my day I often provide hints, tips, and a hand up to those I encounter. I do not do it so they will feel they owe me. I do not want them to feel they owe me. I do want them to appreciate but not so much appreciate me as the fact that we live in a world where help can come to us from a vast number of resources. I want them to feel the abundance that surrounds us in this way. I also do this for a very selfish reason, which is because it makes me feel good when I help others. My personal excitement, pleasure, and satisfaction from uplifting or inspiring another is the greatest gift I could receive. If they do not receive my gift, I don't get mine—the pleasure of knowing I was helpful to someone.

If someone receives my gift and feels gratitude using definition 1 or 2, she will need help again. How much have I truly helped her? She doesn't feel the sense of empowerment someone in a pure state of appreciation feels. She isn't receiving the health and wellbeing benefits that come from being empowered.

Pay attention to your words. Small differences make a difference. When I said that simple changes change your world I meant it. There is a tremendous difference between, "I think I can" and "I can" just as there's a difference between "I'm grateful" and "I appreciate your help." Use your EGS to feel for the differences, and become more attuned to them. It will change how you approach the situation and how you think about it.

Consider your Resources

This process is helpful in emotional stances below the Hopeful Zone. As you pay more attention to how you feel, subtle differences will be more apparent to you. As your chronic emotional stance moves up the EGSc, you will notice if you are below your normal level. When you are, don't panic. Be easy on yourself. Often your resources are depleted. Ask yourself some self-evaluative questions:

- Am I hungry?
- Am I overtired?
- Am I time-stressed?
- Am I in pain?
- Am I worried about something?

When your resources are depleted, you may revert to old habits. Don't worry that you are regressing. Identify what has depleted your resources and, if possible, do something about it. If it is a chronic issue, try to find a way to correct the problem.

When your resources are depleted, it can be difficult to maintain your resolve to attain certain goals. Perhaps you have committed to a new exercise routine but you're so tired that driving to the gym might be an unwise decision. Maybe you can have a salad with some protein for dinner instead of the larger meal you would have chosen. Mix and match things that continue to move you toward your goal. If you are just so exhausted that you can't seem to find the willpower to do anything toward your goal, focus on letting go of stress—which includes not beating yourself up for not doing anything that day. Remember, the self-induced stress from beating yourself up is worse for you than skipping a planned session at the gym.

When you set goals, plan for contingencies. Don't plan your goal as if every single day is going to be as smooth and perfect as you would wish it to be. We, our children, our spouses, and our parents can get sick. There are traffic jams, snow storms, and countless other events that we need to consider when setting goals. Find a balance that works for you. If you're a single parent with one child you might not need as much flexibility as the single parent with two kids. The adult with no children at home might be able to get by with less flexibility built into the plan, unless her parents have health issues or her grown children have grandbabies that might interrupt a plan.

Be flexible in your plans and easy on yourself when your plans stray from the original course. Becoming too stressed about sticking to an inflexible plan increases the stress level when the plan goes awry.

End Self-criticism

The Make Play OK™ Campaign section has several suggestions and examples of how to reduce self-criticism.

The first step to ending self-criticism is to give yourself permission and then set your intentions. For many of us, we have lived with that negative voice in our heads so long we mistake it for who we are. It isn't. It might be your mother, but it isn't your mother when she was in the Sweet Zone. (And yes, it is possible your mother was never in the sweet zone—the possibility of this is a common question in my programs.)

If you do not make much progress eliminating the critic at first, put this intention aside and focus on building your trust in your guidance. Once you have experimented with your guidance and built trust in your answers this task becomes easier. You can use your guidance to ask if what your critic is saying is true, if it is beneficial, and other questions you may have about the inner critic.

When you are ready, refute the comments the inner critic is sharing. If the critic told me I couldn't do something, my response was "Watch me." If the critic told me I wasn't good enough, my response was to find evidence in the world that contradicted the critic. For example, if the critic told me I was unattractive, I would remember times when real people told me the opposite. If the critic told me I wasn't smart enough, I remembered how I have used my brain to solve problems.

You can decide to change something about yourself without declaring your current state of being as bad or unworthy. You are like your life, a journey, not a destination. You are constantly changing and improvements can be part of that journey. There is not a requirement to declare that who you are is bad or wrong in order to grow. Does the crawling infant declare itself bad for not yet walking? No. The same holds true throughout life. You are where you are. Wherever that is can be improved.

Being kind to yourself matters. Do it.

> *"The person in life that you will always be with the most, is yourself. Because even when you are with others, you are still with yourself, too! When you wake up in the morning, you are with yourself, lying in bed at night you are with yourself, walking down the street in the sunlight you are with yourself. What kind of person do you want to walk down the street with? What kind of person do you want to wake up in the morning with? What kind of person do you want to see at the end of the day before you fall asleep? Because that person is yourself, and it's your responsibility to be that person you want to be with. I know I want to spend my life with a person who knows how to let things go, who's not full of hate, who's able to smile and be carefree. So that's who I have to be."*
> — C. JoyBell C.

Low self-esteem usually has one of two roots. One is a habit of comparing oneself to others and looking for flaws. Remember, you are comparing your bloopers to someone else's highlight reel. Don't do that. It is not helpful to you. It does not make you more motivated.

If you're comparing your income to what someone else makes and finding fault with your results, you may also be hastening ill health and an early demise on yourself. There is significant research indicating it is the comparison you make, not the lower income that causes less desirable health outcomes. You can adopt a different perspective. How about, "I'm smarter than he is. If he can make that much, so can I.[127]"

The other common root cause of low self-esteem is a parent or other significant influencer (sometimes a spouse) who repeatedly does and says things to make you feel less than you are. Remember what you have learned about the impact of ES on behavior. No one who was tearing you down was in a good emotional state. Someone in a good emotional state can find something to praise and love about anyone. Their comments, as hurtful as they felt at the time, only contain the power you gave them to hurt you. If you recognize that the comment reflects the person's ES at the time rather than a valid judgment of your worth, the pain lessens.

> *There is nothing noble about being superior to some other man. The true nobility is in being superior to your previous self.*
> Hindu Proverb

While teaching human thriving in high schools, I have had children ask me if it is possible their mom or dad has been angry their whole life. The relief on their face when I said yes let me know I mattered. I would also go on to explain that most people stay in their dominant ES for long periods—often for life—because society has not taught them how to change their ES. Even with the Think Positive movement, the concept was pushed but the how has been largely ignored.

Reframing prior experiences with an understanding that adverse behavior from others was evidence of their low ES and not of your worth can be very healing. It also increases compassion.

Imagine a rebellious teenage girl who has been frequently unkind to her chronically angry, or chronically frustrated, Mother, the epitome of a relationship on a downward spiral without a good ending. The angry Mom is literally training those around them to treat her in ways that make her angry. The daughter has learned this well. Even though she is a good person, without a deliberate intention to be otherwise, she is sucked into the Mom's current of anger. But now, armed with the information that her Mom's behavior is the result of not feeling emotionally good, she can set a new intention. She can decide who she is. For example, she can decide, "I am a kind person. I will do my best to be a positive force in this world." It will take practice because by this time the daughter has developed some neurological pathways that will work against her (just in beginning—later the neurological pathways will help her maintain who she has decided to be).

She can be conscious during her interactions with her mom and when her mom is not being supportive, rather than becoming defensive, she can recognize that her mom is feeling emotionally bad. Armed with that knowledge, she can look for ways to uplift mom—which is the only thing that is going to improve the undesired behavior. In saying this, recognize it is not the teenager's job to uplift her mom. It is not her responsibility. But, unless her mom understands the EGS, the other choices are not good ones. We can ignore mom; however, for a teenager living in her mom's home, this could lead to worsening behavior.

Without an understanding of the EGS, the teenager typically allows an inner critic to move into her mind and suffers low self-esteem that limits her life. With an understand of the EGS, a much better outcome is possible.

My inner critic moved away a few years ago. You can encourage yours to move, too. Humor can help with the persistent inner critic. You can begin telling the critic how nice it is in some place far way, maybe Tahiti, and encouraging it to relocate and that you'll accept four critical postcards a year. Have fun with it. You give the critic its power by believing it. At any time, you have the ability to overthrow its reign.

Oh, and if it is your mom? Don't tell her. It won't help your relationship. It also does not mean she was a bad mom. We live in an era when we have been trained to criticize those we love the most of all. The intention was good. Appreciate that you are learning a better way.

Refute

Refuting is an especially powerful process for anyone who has never questioned his thoughts before. Thoughts do not equate to truth. It is common for someone to have a mistaken impression about someone—leaning too good or too bad.

When we realize that we can decide whether we want to go along with a thought or not, it is empowering. When combined with the EGS we can determine whether a thought is leaning toward truth or not. When the thought feels bad, it is not our truth. When it feels good, it is our truth.

Use your EGS to identify thoughts that are not serving you. When you find one, refute it. Look for evidence of reasons it is wrong.

For example, many people have a belief that goes like this, "Life is hard." If you look at the lives of people with that belief, life is hard for them—but there are many people whose lives are not hard. The belief, "Life is hard" is refutable. Because life is not hard for everyone, you know it is a belief and not destiny. Well, it is destiny if you keep the belief. Refuting it is one way to loosen the belief—sort of like wiggling a loose tooth. The best way to replace beliefs that do not serve you is to overwrite them with better beliefs that do.

If I had this belief (I don't because my life is not hard), I would begin by shifting to a belief along the lines of "Life is hard for some people but I'm learning new skills and it isn't going to be hard for me anymore." I would use this to refute the belief and reinforce the new, more desirable belief.

This would not be my final stop. After I had firmly shifted from "Life is hard" to "Life is hard for some people but I'm learning new skills and it isn't going to be hard for me anymore," I would shift to an even better belief.

Eventually, I would move to the belief: "Life is easy and fun. I live a blessed life."

Remember, the negative emotion you feel when you think a thought that does not serve you means that thought is not the best perspective you can have on that subject. I like to call my thoughts like that "Bogus." It just feels good and lessens the power of those leftover beliefs that are not serving my highest good.

Use Role Models

There is significant evidence that a single good role model can help an otherwise disadvantaged child thrive.

Why does a role model matter?

A role models help children believe in themselves.

Because the role model demonstrates mindsets and thought processes that lead to beneficial outcomes.

This research has led to many programs that match underprivileged children with role models. Such programs are expensive, which means not every child who would benefit from a role model receives one. There is another way, one that is not limited by budgetary constraints.

Anyone can look for examples of role models to help expand his belief in his own potential. Highly successful people are not any better than you are. They have developed supportive patterns of thought. Even IQ is not static[128].

Role models do not have to still be alive and they can even be imaginary. Role models can be in books, movies, video games, or people we actually meet. Look for examples of role models to help you expend your belief in your potential. What do you want for yourself?

Do you want to love fearlessly? Look for examples of individuals who love in that way. It can be in a romantic relationship, familial relationship, or someone who loves others so much he gives his life serving them in some way.

Do you want to maintain your good health into your 80's, 90's or beyond? There are many examples of individuals who are achieving that goal today. Find them and use their success to shore up your belief in your own ability to maintain your vitality beyond the average.

Do you want fame? Success? Creative genius? Your goal does not matter. Believing in your ability to achieve your goal does, and finding others who've achieved those goals gives you more trust in your own abilities. Your EGS will provide you with guidance, but role models of your own choosing will help you adjust your filters. Your EGS will always provide guidance along the shortest path to your goals, but your interpretation of the guidance is more likely to be on target when the programming of your filters is not creating crosswinds.

There is an Irish blessing that begins, *"May the road rise up to meet you. May the wind be always at your back..."* When your beliefs, expectations, emotional stance, and focus are aligned with your goals, following your guidance feels natural (and occurs intuitively). Life feels easier, as if the wind is at your back.

Stop Catastrophizing

Catastrophizing is essentially using a small situation to paint a big catastrophic picture of your world. It is the opposite of using Positive Affirmations. It is affirming what you do not want in a big way.

When someone catastrophizes, they use one incident to decide something about something much bigger than the single incident. For example, failing to complete a project on time at work is failing with one project, one time. It does not make the person a failure.

If you find your emotions spiraling downward, you may be catastrophizing. Stop and think. Stop and feel your EGS. It is not going to agree with your catastrophizing conclusions. Use your EGS and the EGSc to work your way back up the scale.

Catastrophizing is one of the main types of thinking that lead to depression. Set an intention to be more aware of when your thoughts are catastrophizing. When you become aware you are doing this, you're more than half way to stopping it.

Catastrophizing thoughts are not true. They are a way of looking at situations that makes them seem like bigger problems than they are—often they feel dramatic.

If you can't find thoughts on the subject that feel less catastrophic, ask a friend to help you identify new ways of looking at the situation that feel better.

Use Big Picture Perspective to Prevent Arguments

Remember in the Chapter on Beliefs, Expectations, Emotional Stance, and Focus when we discussed mirror neurons and how brains sync to the more dominant point of view? This research is in the early stages, but we have been experimenting with utilizing it as an argument alternative. I am not referring to big picture arguments in realms like religion and politics. It is more the day-to-day arguments and frustrations that we have been experimenting with. For example, take a situation where you and your spouse are going to landscape your yard. As you discuss the plans, you learn that the vision your partner has differs from what you want, and you really want it to be your way. The old-fashioned way is to argue about it until one of you is weary of arguing and gives in.

In the Mirror Sync alternative, ignore what your spouse wants and focus exclusively on the vision you have of your yard. Imagine every nuance of the way it will look when it is complete. Imagine going outside and seeing it complete, how it will look and how it will feel.

The brains sync to the one with the most dominant thoughts on the subject. This process focuses your mind on what you want, making your vision dominant.

Think back to the chapter on Coherent Thoughts. What is happening in an argument? You think a thought that is lined up with your goals (coherence) then you think about what your partner wants and how it differs from what you want (destructive interference). This is why arguments are so unproductive—neither brain is establishing a dominant position.

There is an even larger benefit coming out of our experiments with this process. We are finding that, as we shore up our own belief to make it more dominant, we find a flaw in our thought process that was creating the discord in the first place. The disagreement is solved because we see something we miscalculated.

For example, in the visions of your landscaping, you might have ignored the necessity of moving the lawnmower from the front yard to the back yard. As you spend time visualizing what you want, the flaw becomes apparent to you. At that point, you adjust your vision to correct the flaw, bringing your vision closer to that of your spouse.

When you argue against what you do not want, you are visualizing what you do not want instead of what you want. The destructive interference on the quantum level ensures this is unproductive.

When the initial disagreement occurs there is stress involved. Taking a step back to focus on what you want not only gives more power to your side of the argument, it reduces your stress and, once you feel better, it's easy to see that your desires don't include arguments with those you love. This tool is specifically good for arguments, but try visualizing how you want your day to turn out before you get out of bed (when you're in a good head space) and see how much better things can be.

Breathe

For most of us, breathing is something we do without thought. But breathing consciously can be very comforting. Place a note somewhere you will see it often. Write Breathe[129] on the note. When you see the note, consciously take a deep slow breathe in and then release. Repeat as necessary until you feel calmer. If you know you are going to have a stressful day, you can set reminders to pop-up on your computer or smart phone reminding you to breathe.

This process is recommended for any zone below the Hopeful Zone. It can provide immediate releasing of stress. Long-term benefits are possible if deeper, more conscious breathing becomes a habit.

Handling Difficult Times

This process makes some suggestions for changing your mindset during times that we often perceive as difficult. We'll use a Mother/Son relationship for our example. Suppose your son is somewhere that feels dangerous to you and you do not want him to be there. You have no control over the situation. Your son could be in prison or in a military war zone. If you suffer by thinking about him and about all that could befall him, you are spending your days suffering but your worry does not help him one iota. It does not keep him safer. It does not bring him back sooner. It only diminishes the life you are leading. It diminishes your happiness, which diminishes your own well-being. This makes you less able to be there for him when he returns. It depletes your psychological reserves. Both worry and love are emotions. You can only do one or the other at any given moment in time. Your emotional feedback system is sending you the emotion of love or the emotion of worry in response to your thoughts. You are not receiving both at the same time.

If you choose to focus on loving him, you will be inspired with ideas about how you can love him while he is there. Perhaps you will keep a journal of appreciation about him in which you record thoughts you have of love and things you appreciate and admire about him. Wouldn't that be a lovely gift to give him when he returns? If the loved one has the ability to receive letters, you could mail snippets to him. Compare a letter of love and appreciation to one of worry. The first would uplift while the second could inspire guilt and concern on his part. If your son is in a war zone (and I would consider both examples to be exactly that) you want him to focus the best he can. The better he feels, the better he is able to do this. The Broaden and Build Theory[130] has clearly demonstrated this.

What is the Broaden and Build Theory? It is research by Barbara L. Fredrickson, Ph.D. into the benefits of positivity. One aspect of positivity she was able to demonstrate is that we have increased cognitive abilities when we feel good.

How do you not worry? At first, you have to make a conscious choice that your intention is to do your best for your son and yourself. Consciously recognize that the choice is to love him and acknowledge that worry is not love. In your worry, you intend to love, but in the moments when you are worrying, you are not loving. We only experience one emotion at a time even though we can feel that we are experiencing more than one at a time because emotions can change very quickly. We are not.

We experience an emotion in response to a thought and as we think another thought, another emotion (or the same one) is felt in response to the thought.

So, first make the decision to love. Then your mind (helped by the filters you have now set with this deliberate intention) begins thinking thoughts about to show love to a loved one who is far away. Ideas come to you that support that decision. As the ideas flow, act upon them.

As you work on the project, you think about your son, as he was then, safe and loved. In doing so, you flow that love to him energetically and your own well-being is increased.

Many people might encourage you to worry. They might say that is what a good parent would do in those circumstances. Do they know that your worry is not healthy for you and does nothing for your child? Do they know that your decision to love makes you stronger and has the potential to benefit your child? Just because most people in that situation worry does not mean it is the right decision. You have the right to make decisions that feel best to you. There is no requirement that you do as others do in like circumstances. You are a thinking sentient being capable of making your own decisions.

If it makes it easier, do not tell them how happy you are. Or, if it feels better, tell them and confound them.

If your sister says, "How can you seem so happy when your son is in the war zone?" you can respond, "I think about him often and about how much I love him. I can't wait to see him when he comes home. I can savor the joy of his homecoming now and I do it often."

Unable to see your perspective, your sister says, "Aren't you worried you'll be disappointed if something happens?"

You do not allow her to upset your confidence, "Why would I think anything would happen? Most people come home from the war just fine. Why would I think my son would be an exception?"

Your sister clings to her worrisome position, "You are asking for trouble with your confidence."

Recognizing that she has an underlying belief that is not serving her, which would not serve you, you stand your ground, "No, I am loving my son; just as he is, where he is. When he comes home our relationship will be better than ever because I am learning to love him unconditionally while he is away."

Confused, your sister asks, "How can you love him unconditionally? What if he does something you don't want him to do?"

You can respond, "It is his life to do with as he pleases. If I make my happiness contingent on his decisions, I give him the power to decide if I will be happy or not. I will not give that power away. Now that I know the truth of happiness, I am not giving my power away again."

Your Sister may or may not ever understand your position but I hope the example helps you see that it does not matter. You can choose to be happy regardless of what anyone else feels about that decision. Any other decision gives your power away to other people. You do not need the permission of another to be happy. Happiness is a personal choice.

Chapter 17: Processes (How to Think Positive)

Chapter 18: Permission to Self

Beliefs have the power to create and the power to destroy. Human beings have the awesome ability to take any experience of their lives and create a meaning that disempowers them or one that can literally save their lives.

Tony Robbins

Happiness Contracts

Each individual has developed beliefs about happiness. In *Be Happy*, Dr. Robert Holden[131] wrioted "Your Happiness Contract asserts every condition, rule, and law that you absolutely must abide by in order to be eligible for any amount of happiness. Any happiness that you experience without first fulfilling these conditions is strictly 'illegal' and may result in personal penalties of guilty feelings, inner discomfort, and moral foreboding."

Your personal happiness contract is the result of the way you perceive the life experiences you have lived. If you had to be good for Santa Claus to bring you the much desired toy, you probably have a requirement to "be good" in your happiness contract.

The truth is that happiness is your right. Happiness is free. There are no dues, no conditions, and no ways to earn happiness.

I discuss some common beliefs about happiness that are in many happiness contracts to help you identify and eradicate any conditions that are hindering your ability to be happy.

I suggest adopting a **happiness contract** as follows:

> I deserve to be happy. When I am happy, I am at my best. I am in the best health. I am in the best mood. I am able to think with greater clarity. I am able to see solutions to problems far more readily. I need less from others (pumping up, assistance of all types, etc.). I contribute more by being happy so being happy is a

priority for me. When I am happy, I contribute to others by inspiring them to happiness. I contribute to others because when I feel great I want to help others feel just as wonderful. Sometimes when someone feels rotten, it makes her feel better to see someone else who feels rotten, or see someone who is even worse off than she is. When I am happy, it lifts me even higher to help others up and I gain no happiness or relief from their not being in a good place. When I am happy, seeing others succeed reminds me that I am capable and if they can do it, it is possible for me. Minding my happiness is minding my health because when I am happy I am inclined to make good decisions about my diet, exercise, and other habits. Happiness reduces stress on my body and enables it to maintain its health with ease. My happiness is good for me and good for the world.

Some false premises about happiness are provided below to help you identify your current happiness contract and decide if you want to reprogram your beliefs about happiness:

False Premise about Happiness #1: *I have to be perfect before I deserve happiness.*

This is completely bogus. No one and everyone is perfect.

Everyone is perfect because everyone is the best they can be in every moment. We are human. We are not a work of art like Michelangelo's David, unchanging through time. We are works of art in progress and our goal is to enjoy the journey, not to rush to the destination. In every moment, there is a way to perceive our circumstances that serves our highest good. Each time we reach a goal, new ones appear. Savoring the journey is the only way to enjoy life.

> *Not seeking your personal happiness has a greater chance of making you a burden to society.*

In moments when things feel perfect, we are savoring the fruits of our labor. In moments when things feel less than perfect we are learning and growing and further defining our destination by learning what is not desired.

False Premise about Happiness #2: *I must sacrifice good things for happiness.*

This is based on the false premise that seeking personal happiness is selfish and therefore wrong. The happiness contract suggested above reflects many reasons why selfishly seeking happiness for yourself is good for you, and also good for the world.

I love Dr. Holden's words and suggestion that if you must sacrifice, you sacrifice "fear for love, guilt for joy" and I would add jealousy for appreciation, unworthiness for worthiness, powerlessness for empowerment, contentment for positive expectation, boredom for enthusiasm, despair for positive expectation, stress for equanimity, sickness for health, and pessimism for optimism.

The belief that sacrifice is required before happiness is deserved is often the result of feelings of unworthiness. Entire manuscripts have been written on this subject. However, the EGS is a fantastic tool for this task. The most important thing anyone can do to improve self-esteem is to stop self-criticism. The positive feedback the EGS provides gives clear evidence that tearing yourself down is not on your path toward self-realization. You will achieve more in every area of life by being emotionally supportive of your dreams.

False Premise about Happiness #3: *Happiness must be earned.*

While a good work ethic is fine and valuable, a work ethic fueled by passion and enthusiasm for the tasks at hand is far superior to a work ethic fueled by a carrot on a stick, which is what this is.

This belief is leftover from an old paradigm that is not supported by science. When this belief is brought out into the light of day, it is easy to see the fallacy of this belief. Science has been proving that success does not make one happy; many people society defines as successful are unhappy in important areas of their lives.

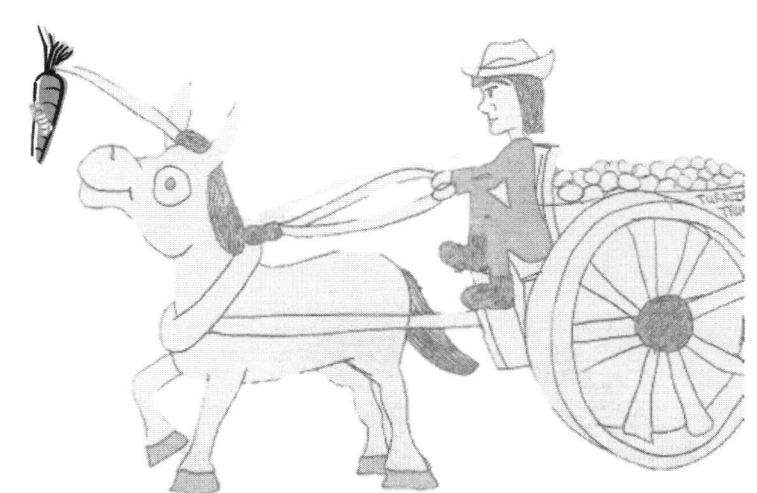

I do not intend to imply that people who believe this false premise are stupid, merely that they have not examined their beliefs against how the world really works. They are living under an old paradigm that believed happiness resulted from hard work and success.

That belief does not reflect reality. Individuals who are positively focused achieve far greater success throughout life—in every area of life—than those who are not positively focused. Being happy first increases one's success in marriage, in health, in work, and in relationships.

When I look at an old way of viewing happiness, I ask myself, who would benefit from this belief? Someone, and not the person chasing the stick, benefited from this paradigm.

In third world countries, many individuals who live in conditions we would find abhorrent are happier than many of us who live in relative luxury. Happiness is not earned; it is about perspective.

If you focus your attention on allowing yourself to be happy, the other aspects of your life will fall more easily into place. Happiness includes following your dreams. Aren't good relationships, successful careers, and good health part of our dreams? We want meaningful work and we want to do a good job toward that meaningful goal. Our emotional guidance guides us towards realization of all our goals.

False Premise about Happiness #4: *You cannot know happiness unless you have suffered and sacrificed.*

This is not true. Look at the babies. Babies know happiness and have not suffered.

You cannot sacrifice enough to make yourself happy. Happiness is a birthright of every individual. The belief that you have to sacrifice to know happiness is a learned belief that we have to do something in order to be happy. When we are our authentic selves and love who we are, we can be happy now.

Suffering is unnatural and we should not suffer. Suffering does not add to the world. Your suffering does not make the world a better place. Your happiness makes the world a better place.

> *If you're stressing over happiness, you are doing it wrong!*
> *Shannon L. Alder*

False Premise about Happiness #5: *Happiness will be punished.*

In many cases, this becomes a self-fulfilling prophecy. Those who believe it and wait for "the other shoe to drop" use fear of what may happen in the future to destroy the present. This belief causes you to look for problems, setting the filters in your mind to see problems and not the good.

There are no angry or jealous gods as the ancient Greek and Roman myths talk about. Humans are not punished for being happy. If you see evidence in the world of individuals who were happy and then not happy, they probably had this expectation. Their focus on what could go wrong caused them to find things to fuss and worry about until they were no longer happy.

Set an intention to look for individuals who have been happy for a long time. When you find examples, use those examples to strengthen your knowledge that there is no balloon payment due on your happiness, no toll for traveling that road.

False Premise about Happiness #6: *I must be enlightened to know real happiness.*

This is like the belief that success will result in happiness. When we are happy first, enlightenment becomes much easier to achieve. When you choose to be happy, you are more in tune with your true self.

Remember, the babies and little ones. Spend time watching them. Notice how easily they return to happiness even when they were crying moments before. There they are now, laughing, with the tears not yet dry on their faces.

We do not have to learn how to be happy. We remember how to be happy.

It is about letting go of things that do not feel good and holding onto those things that do feel good.

Think about one of your happiest moments. Remember how alive you felt? Remember how much stronger and more vital you felt at those times? Remember how the world suddenly seemed a better place? Let your thoughts flow toward those thoughts—that you are strong, vital, and deliciously alive. Feel your love for the beauty of this world. Feel your love for those with whom you share this world.

Now, that feels far more enlightened than thoughts of having to "find" happiness or seek enlightenment in order to be happy. You see, it is right there for you to have now, in this moment.

Happiness is your natural state. When you are happy, you have a closer connection to all things. Happiness is the key to enlightenment.

False Premise about Happiness #7: *Everyone must agree that I deserve happiness before it is okay for me to be happy.*

Have you ever tried to get 100% approval for anything from more than one other person?

This belief will surely set you up for failure.

It is also bogus.

Why should another's beliefs and expectations impact your ability to be happy? Why is another's perception more valid than your own? Does any other person even spend enough time to really know your true situation or your thoughts, ideas and beliefs to be able to make this decision for you? Not even your mother gives you this much attention after the first few months. No one can. Everyone is focused on self, seeing the world from a unique personal perspective. When someone else wants you to do something (go to college, become a lawyer, marry a certain individual, marry at all, etc.), they are really expressing what would make them happy which may have nothing at all to do with what would make you happy. Their job is not to make you happy and your job is not to make them happy. Our job is to learn how to be happy regardless of what others choose to do. That is freedom and that is unconditional love.

When you are being who you think someone else wants you to be, you will probably expect them to be who you want them to be. Doesn't that sound confining? Think of the freedom in being who you really are. Doesn't it feel good to give others that same freedom? Much of the friction that exists in relationships is from feeling as if you are bound into a mold that does not fit well anymore. This can come about in so many ways. It can come because we mistakenly tried to be who we thought they wanted us to be in the beginning and now we are stuck in that role. Or it could be that we were who we really are in the beginning but they expect us to be unchanging when our very nature is to change continually and grow and expand who we are becoming.

You can lose track of who you really are when you try to be someone different to please another. Choose to be true to who you really are; both you and others will get the best of you.

Some fear that if we are true to who we are we will not be good but that is another false premise. When we are at the high end of the EGSc what we give others is good. Only people who feel trapped at the lower ends of the EGSc exhibit abhorrent behavior. It is not possible to stay at the high levels of the EGSc unless you are being who you really are.

When my daughter made her school decisions and I found the positive aspects of each of the decisions I was choosing to love her unconditionally. Her decision had no bearing on my love for her nor did it have any bearing on my ability to be happy because I have learned how to be happy regardless of what others choose to do. I do not give others control of whether or not I can be happy.

You can choose to be happy regardless of what anyone else feels about that decision. Any other decision gives your power away to that other (or those other) people. You do not need the permission of another to be happy. Happiness is a personal choice.

It is also not necessary for others to be happy before you can be happy. If you wait for everyone else to be happy, you may wait forever.

False Premise about Happiness #8: *I must have control of my circumstances before I can be happy.*

This is another path to a never-ending search for happiness. There are too many moving parts for anyone to control their circumstances fully. You cannot control even one other person without putting yourself into bondage in your requirement to make sure the other follows all your instructions. The aspects of the world that are beyond your control are too many to even begin listing them all, but they would include politics, the weather, the economy, behavior, opinions and decisions of others, and so on. You get the idea.

Your happiness is about your perception and how you react to the circumstances—It is not about controlling circumstances.

Loving the people in your life unconditionally is a good way to let go of the need to control them. You can even decide to love them even if their behavior is such that you no longer want to spend time with them. You do not have to stop loving them to decide you do not want to spend time with them. The decisions are best kept mutually exclusive.

If you learn to love unconditionally, you will not have a lack of wonderful people in your life.

Looking for the positive aspects in each situation helps you give up the need to control. You can choose happiness regardless of conditions.

Happiness is about choosing to be who you really are, not about requiring others or circumstances to be whom and what you want them to be. When you are true to who you really are, you do not require others to be different in order to please you.

False Premise about Happiness #9: *I have to be completely independent in order to be happy.*

While it is wonderful to know that you have the ability to be self-sufficient, many individuals insist on repeatedly proving it long after they have demonstrated their ability.

Think about how you feel when you know someone you care about is in need. Doesn't it feel good to do something for them? Lending a shoulder to cry on, fixing chicken noodle soup, introducing connections that can help a friend find a job, and other helpful actions can make the giver feel good. When actions are taken because the individual wants to help, allowing the person to help is a gift. Many people reject help that is proffered because they do not want to feel indebted, not realizing allowing help may be giving a gift. It feels good to be in a position where you can do for those you care about.

Would you deprive your friends and loved ones of the opportunity to do those things for you that you would gladly do for them? Asking for and receiving help does not diminish your value. Studies have shown that too much independence weakens us.

The world is a community and there are many who will feel joy at helping others. If you are in a position where you need help, ask for it and let it come to you.

Often when someone helps another, things that are far more valuable to the person than what was given are learned. There is something about helping another who you help because you want to that gets you into those high places on the EGS where epiphany's seem to flow easily.

If you find yourself in need of help, accept it but also accept responsibility for where you are and how you got there. There is great power in accepting responsibility. If you are responsible for where you are, you have the ability to move forward. If you blame your circumstances on others, you feel powerless in the world. Appreciate the help that you receive.

Also, remember that what may seem like a negative life event often ends up being "the best thing that ever happened to you" in hindsight after you have moved through the experience.

- The lay-off of a good job leads to a better job that you would not have even looked for if not for the lay-off.
- The spouse who leaves you makes room for the love of your life to walk into your life.
- The dire diagnosis gives you a new zest for life and new perspectives that enrich your life in ways that would never have happened without that event.
- The business failure brings forth the knowledge that makes the next business far more successful than it would have been without the prior failure.
- Losing the game inspires greater desire that creates a world-class athlete.

The world is full of examples of those who thought at the time that an event was "the end of the world" who later appreciate the gifts from that event. If your own life has not shown this to you, there are two ways to firm up this belief. One is to look back at past events, briefly, to see if they have not given you gifts that you have not consciously recognized. Another is to read the stories of those whose lives have demonstrated this clearly.

False Premise about Happiness #10: *I must be good before I can be happy.*

In countries that celebrate Christmas with Santa Claus, the idea that only good little boys and girls get the presents has potential to set the stage for internalizing this belief. Parents who require a child to be good in order to receive a reward that provides temporary happiness is another way this concept is commonly reinforced.

The truth is that every person is as good as he or she can be in each moment. Their position on the EGSc determines how good their best in that moment is, but no one wakes up and says, "I am going to be less than my best today." It feels best to do our best in every moment even when our best in that moment is not our best possible or best ever.

This is an arbitrary standard. What is good? Who is going to define that?

When you are at the high end of the EGSc what you give the world is wonderful and it is because that is what you feel like giving. When you are lower on the EGS *trying* to be good, it often feels like a struggle. Therefore, choosing happiness allows you to be your best easily. There is nothing wrong with easy. It does not have to be a struggle and there is no added value in making it a struggle.

When you choose happiness first, your goodness is a natural part of who you are.

False Premise about Happiness #11: *Too much happiness will change me and that makes me afraid.*

As you move up the EGSc, your increased happiness will change how you show up in the world, but it will not diminish you or change your true nature.

True happiness will allow your true nature to shine forth from within.

The truth is that we all change all the time. What do you want to change into? More of the same or the best you can be?

There are risks. Friends and family with whom your relationship is based upon shared places at the lower ends of the EGSc may become less prominent in your life, or less enjoyable. Do you want to hold yourself in a place that is less than where you could be because others are there? You can choose to be the leader and lead by your example inspiring them to feel better too (but wait until you are stable in the new place before you do this).

The higher you are on the EGSc, the more people will want to be around you. You will be a magnet to others who want what you have found. While you have no responsibility to help another be happy, it can be great fun to do so when the other is ready.

What clauses do you have in your happiness contract? Do you feel like you could let go of those conditions to being happy? What are the benefits of removing those pre-conditions?

False Premise about Happiness #12: *Happiness is about materialism.*

True happiness has nothing to do with materialism. Material goods are neither the cause of happiness nor the cause of unhappiness. The way you perceive material goods can cause happiness or unhappiness. In fact, the split between material and spiritual is recent and a construct created by man[132] when the Cartesian Split between science and religion, leaving the mind to religion occurred.

If you have something you see as desired and valuable, you feel happy when you focus on it. Then, if you have beliefs that you have to "keep up with Joneses," when your neighbor gets something you perceive as better than what you have, you make yourself unhappy by accepting the perception that what your neighbor has is better than what you have.

You have the ability to change your perception in ways that make you happier without requiring the purchase of something you may not really want. Find a perception about what you already own that feels better than the one that concludes what your neighbor has is better. Examples:

- "Mine is perfectly good and by being happy with this one, I will be able to afford a vacation with my family this year."

- "Mine serves its purpose and I am more relaxed not going into debt to buy a new car."
- "I am lucky. My things always last longer than others' things do."
- "I don't have to impress anyone else. They don't know everything about me and if they think my being older means I am less than Mr. Jones, that is their problem."
- "The people in my life who matter love me for who I am, not what I own."

What examples can you come up with that will help you not feel envious of others? Envy really comes from an underlying belief that you cannot have what the other person has. When you believe you can have what another is able to have, it inspires you.

Many people have constructed beliefs about how good they are based on a foundation of having things that are as good as, or better than, what others have. This makes their happiness contingent on staying ahead. It is the belief, not the nature of happiness, that bundles happiness and materialism. Eliminating the belief that your possessions have anything to do with your value or worth will free you from one common tie between happiness and materialism. There is nothing wrong with wanting material goods, but attaching your worthiness to your possessions is harmful to your wellbeing. Unbundling your worth from your possessions helps you make better decisions about what to acquire and decisions are more likely to be driven by true desires, instead of perceived competition with someone else.

Some people who have great wealth are unhappy. Some people living in dire circumstances are happy. Many years ago I traveled to St. Lucia and found the people there to be some of the happiest I had ever encountered despite the fact that most of them lived in sheds that were worse than I kept my lawn mower in. I was confused by this at the time. Now I understand that material possessions have nothing to do with creating happiness. When we make happiness about obtaining material possessions, it decreases our happiness.

False Premise about Happiness #13: *It is more important to be right (and never be shown to have been wrong) than to be happy.*

We hold onto our personal opinions and beliefs because we believe they define who we are. When we begin understanding how our brain proves our beliefs to us, making them true for us, the motivation to change beliefs that do not serve our highest good becomes stronger than our desire to have been right in the past. If defending the belief does not move us toward our highest good, adopting new beliefs that support self-realization feels more important than defending what we used to believe.

This is a short-term view that sabotages longer-term goals. It leads to the Galileo Effect and, on the personal level, to less harmonious relationships.

Although I recommend a happiness contract that I believe will serve you well, you get to choose what is right for you. My hope is that your choice will help you be all that you dream of becoming. Remember:

> In your state of happiness, you have sereneness about you that others find pleasurable, comforting, and calming to be around. Often, once you choose happiness and become stable in that zone, others will ask you how you have done it. From a position of happiness you can encourage and inspire others to happiness, not because you are saying "I need you to be happy in order for me to be happy," but because they see how you are doing and want to come to have what you have achieved. You can't push others to happy when you are trying from a state of unhappiness in order to get them happy so it will be "okay" for you to be happy but once you are happy you can inspire them to come to where you are because you suddenly seem wiser when you are happy. In their desire to be happy, people will seek "pearls of wisdom" from you. Everyone wants to be happy, even if they have buried the desire so deeply that they are not aware of it.
>
> *Happiness indicates a low level of stress. Either way you view it, increasing happiness or reducing stress, the result is improved health, relationships, success, and well-being.* That may be the most important reason your happiness is good for the world; your unhappiness is not.

Chapter 18: Permission to Self

Chapter 19: A Global Solution

Humanity is asking for a global solution to the health care crisis. The common view is that a solution is not possible because of cost constraints. Not only is a solution possible, it is here. The cost is not too high—it is the cost of not acting now that is too high.

We must turn our attention away from the problems and toward the solution. When we focus on the problem, the solution cannot be seen. The problem tells us what we do not want. We must look at those things that work, as we want all things to work and then move toward replacing the root of the problem with the root of wellbeing. We know the root of wellbeing. The research is clear. Beneath the symptoms, beneath the risk factors, is a common element—that element is stress. It would be difficult to find an illness or social problem without unmanaged stress at its basis.

Our society has to shift some fundamental beliefs. We have grown accustomed to ignoring stress and accepting high levels of stress as normal and tolerable—this acceptance created the healthcare crisis. Fundamental changes in the way we view and address stress are required to stop the escalating emotional and financial burden of disease our world.

The solution is neither expensive nor difficult. We know, but usually ignore, that the way an individual perceives a situation effects how much actual stress that individual experiences. We know the mindset of the individual is the determining factor in how the situation is perceived, which in turn determines how stressful the situation is to them. The actual stress experienced, not the situation, dictates the biochemical responses their body experiences. Those biochemical responses to stress effect health at its basis—the immune function.

The newest research provides the final piece of the puzzle, the one that unlocks the door for humanity to thrive in unprecedented ways. The Emotional Sensory Feedback System will help every individual that learns how to understand its language and to respond to the guidance it provides using Right Responses to avoid diseases that would otherwise manifest due to unmanaged stress. There are also significant benefits beyond health, including increased resilience and emotional intelligence, using the methods described herein. Increasing resilience and emotional intelligence provide a protective effect for many social concerns including alcohol and drug abuse, suicide, other forms of self-harm, and it improves relationships.

We stand before an open door—a door to a level of health and wellbeing most of us have never imagined—a level that will benefit every individual on Earth.

Why is this **the solution**?

Global stress management training is the solution and not just for the obvious reason—that it works. It is also affordable. In fact, globally, I predict that there will be tremendous cost savings due to the improved health and social environments that will result. Teaching individuals to understand the purpose and language of their emotional guidance system does not require a great deal of time or money. Training can be done in large groups. In fact, it is better in large groups so the trainees have others to talk with and compare notes about their experiences. Modern technology makes it even more affordable. Every person has guidance to help them understand how to thrive more.

Positive emotions are both contagious and inspirational. I long ago lost track of how many times I heard "I want your life" from someone I was interacting with. I never heard this before I learned how to use my EGS. My answer is always the same "Yours can be as good or better." I want everyone to have the life they desire, fulfilling as much of their potential as possible.

When healthier and more accurate foundations for our society replace the false premises that create so many of the mindsets that cause high stress and low health outcomes, training will not be necessary. Parents, teachers, and religious leaders will stop teaching our children away from their inborn guidance. The possibilities for the future are so wonderful they seem unbelievable.

Those possibilities extend far beyond greater health and wellbeing. The research demonstrates a behavioral link to emotion. Teaching individuals how to increase their emotional set points will not just confer better health—it will greatly reduce socially undesirable behaviors. The root cause of crime is the same as the root cause of so much poor health—stress. We could begin reducing recidivism now and within a generation, most of the prisons could be empty—not because we decriminalize any behaviors—but because the root cause of crime has been eliminated.

Many mental health issues stem from unhealthy thinking patterns that degenerate into mental health diagnoses. Understanding how we perceive reality combined with greater attention to what we are thinking and the feedback from our EGS will naturally reduce the incidence of mental health issues.

We have to begin looking deeper at our decisions. There is compelling evidence that chronic stress is the most significant contributor to poor health, relationship, success, and wellbeing outcomes. For forty years, reduction of stress has been recommended as prevention, but the root cause has not been addressed.

Science has recently shown that emotions are actually feedback from a sensory feedback system designed to guide us away from harm and toward self-realization. We know one of the main contributors to stress is mindsets that do not support the individual's highest good. The Emotional Guidance Sensory Feedback System provides feedback that helps each individual adjust their mindset to one that more fully supports their unique goals. We have to stop teaching our children to misinterpret the guidance that was designed to help them thrive!

The EGS is self-reinforcing, when an individual understands how to interpret its messages accurately, better-feeling emotions lead the individual toward self-actualization.

The level of stress deemed acceptable by much of the world is the underlying reason for increased incidents of preventable diseases. Reducing stress increases positivity, they are two sides of the same coin. The research must be looked at in total—not in isolation. The combined benefits of decreasing stress and increasing positivity have positive influences on cancers, heart disease, Alzheimer's prevention, immune function, pregnancy outcomes, relationships, success, cognitive function, resilience, emotional intelligence, diabetes, obesity, depression, anxiety, addictions, crime, teen pregnancy, colds, flu, and more.

We stand in front of a door to unprecedented improvements in life on Earth. Humanity deserves the benefits of this knowledge now. We expend significant resources toward the problems that these recommendations will solve. Imagine what else we can do when those resources are redirected to any remaining problems.

Training the world to understand their EGS is a one-time event. It is not something that will have to be repeated with each new generation because parents will teach their children. Societies will be designed understanding that each individual has guidance toward their highest good. The problems that plague classrooms today will be something children read about in history books, not what they experience on a daily basis.

We stand in the doorway of a world so much better for all than the one that exists. Today, we live in a world where nations are willing to enter wars not knowing the price that will ultimately be paid—but will they move toward something good with as much faith in the outcome? Will we hesitate in the doorway, as generations before have done when presented with strong evidence that something was beneficial but all the reasons it worked were not yet known, or will we boldly move forward and provide our children and their children, for generations to come, a better world?

Chapter 19: A Global Solution

Einstein said:

> *"The most important decision we make is whether we believe we live in a friendly or hostile universe."*
>
> *Albert Einstein*

Today we need to decide if we live in a world where there are solutions to our problems or not. Science has been demonstrating the benefits of positivity, increased resilience, increased emotional intelligence, and reduced stress for years. The final piece of the puzzle is in place with the research published in Global Advances in Health and Medicine. It is time to move confidently in the direction of the future we want.

In *Happier*, Tal Ben Shahar wrote, "Blaming others—our parents, our teachers, our boss, or the government—may yield sympathy but not happiness. The ultimate responsibility...lies with us." [133] This program places the responsibility on each individual to master the ability to self-manage his or her own stress level, but that responsibility is aided by intrinsic motivation built into the emotional feedback system.

Will we continue being a world more apt to enter a war with an unknown outcome due to fear or will we overcome the Galileo Effect and claim the world we want for our own?

I think we are smart enough to make the right choice. I think we have the courage and the will to move forward, implementing a program that can help each person thrive more. Think of the legacy we will leave to future generations if we move forward confidently. Compare that to the legacy we leave if we do not. Do we really have a choice?

The generations who went before cannot be blamed. They did not know about the false premises that were undermining their ability to thrive—false premises they passed on to their children with the best of intentions. No, they are not to blame.

We do not have that luxury. We know. If we do not act on what we know, we will be responsible. I don't think we need that negative incentive—I think we are smart enough to move toward creating the world we want because it is the right thing to do and because the research is clear enough that anything less than full motion forward is preposterous.

I mean each person who reads this should take action. Do not just read the book. Experiment with your EGS, use the processes, share the information, talk about it with your friends, your doctor, your political representatives, and especially your children.

Acknowledgments

Without the wisdom of those who came before me, and those who have traveled parts of the road I am now on, my understanding of human thriving would never have reached the level it has. Contributions have come from ancient philosophers to modern physicists, psychologists, physicians, and mystics.

Like droplets of fine wine poured into a glass, once combined, it is impossible to separate them again. As with every student, information I found was given meaning based on the beliefs, expectations, emotional stance, and focus I had at the time. I believe an epiphany occurs when a shift in ones filters allows them to see something in a new, more enlightened way than they previously viewed it. I have experienced many epiphanies during my journey. Does that mean I am especially knowledgeable, or just that I had far to travel? From my own perspective that question cannot be answered. I only know it feels like both.

Every person in my life has influenced my perspective on human thriving, whether in person or via a book. The bibliography includes many whose work provided bits and pieces of the answers my the question, what makes humans thrive?

The support of my family as I worked on this project has been wonderful. The support and encouragement from my fiancée and daughters is warm and supporting.

Disclaimer

I do not know the reader personally and even if I did, I am not a licensed physician so I cannot legally advise you about the best course of action for your unique circumstances. If you are under the care of a physician, I recommend you do not stop that care without the approval of a physician.

However, if your physician does not seem to believe in your potential recovery, or if she insists on advising you in ways that could create a nocebo effect on your health, I encourage you to seek help from a different physician.

I have personally been helped by the advice in this book and seen it help hundreds of others in significant ways. I have seen shifts from suicidal to hopeful in short periods. I have seen excess weight melt away and chronic health conditions improve.

If you believe you are in danger of harming yourself or another, please seek professional help immediately. Learn the processes and gain an understanding of the information in this book in tandem with any care prescribed by your physician. I believe it will speed your recovery and make it more stable than traditional methods of care.

National Suicide Prevention Hotline: 1-800-273-8255

If for any reason the number does not work, please look in your telephone directory, or use a search engine to find the current number.

If you believe you may be depressed or you feel the following symptoms of depression describe you, please contact a licensed professional.

- The pleasure and joy have gone out of my life
- My future seems hopeless
- I have lost interest in things that used to be important to me
- I feel agitated
- Life seems like too much effort
- I am a bad person
- I think about how I could kill myself
- My weight has changed
- It is difficult for me to concentrate
- Making decisions is difficult
- I feel sad, powerless, unhappy
- I am tired all the time
- I am a failure
- I can't sleep well
- I can't see a way out
- Good things do not bring me joy

Send Me Your Stories

I would love to hear how you use the Emotional Guidance System and about epiphanies you experience along the way. Please send your comments, stories, suggestions to: `MyStory@Happiness1st.com`

Thank you. ♥ Jeanine Joy

Feel Inspired to Help?

Anyone who experiments with his or her emotional guidance realizes how much it improves one's life experience. Those who understand that the joy of others benefits everyone may want to help spread these skills. Phil and I have established a non-profit organization, Achieve Affinity. The mission is to bring information & resources to those who would otherwise have limited access to these life-enhancing skills. While learning how to interpret your own EGS and self-manage your emotional stance is a gift to the world and all those with whom you share the planet, many are moved to do more. If you would like to donate time, funds, or other benefits please see our website www.AchieveAffinity.org or mail to:

Achieve Affinity
P.O. Box 6888
Concord NC 28027

Currently, donations are tax-deductible in the USA, please doublecheck with your tax advisor. A non-profit 501(c)(3) organization has been established to bring skills and knowledge that increases thriving to people around the world.

Thank you very much.

Are you a researcher?

We are happy to partner with researchers to demonstrate the increased thriving children and adults experience as a result of the programs. Documenting the benefits opens doors that allow us to bring greater well-being to more people.

Contact us via our websites:

www.Happiness1st.com/programs
www.JeanineJoy.US

or by sending mail to:

Thrive More, Now
P.O. Box 6888
Concord NC 28078

Programs, Retreats, and Cruises

Happiness 1st Institute offers programs to corporations, individuals, and other institutions. Programs are offered in a variety of formats including in-person and on-line programs, retreats, cruises, and executive coaching. CD and DVD programs are in the works. You may reach us through our websites:

```
www.Happiness1st.com
www.Happiness1st.com/programs
```

If you are interested in joining us on an educational and fun cruise, be sure to send us your Email address. We will let you know when we plan the next one.

```
Cruises@Happiness1st.com
```

Be the first to learn about upcoming events and programs by signing up for our Newsletter.

Contact us to see Jeanine Joy's availability for speaking engagements.

Bibliography

n.d. 1 3 2014.
<http://en.wikipedia.org/wiki/United_States_military_casualties_of_war (3/1/2014)>.

Achor, Shawn. *The Happiness Advantage: Seven Principles of Positive Psychology That Fuel Success and Performance at Work.* Random House, 2010.

American Health Association Journals. n.d. 1 3 2014.
<http://circ.ahajournals.org/content/123/4/e18.full>.

Andrews, Robyn A., Roger Lowe and Anne Clair. "The relationship between basic need satisfaction and emotional eating in obesity." *Australian Journal of Psychology* (2011): 207-213.

Armstrong, Andrew R., Roslyn F. Galligan and Christine R. Critchley. "Emotional Intelligence and psychological resilience to negative life events." *Personality and Individual Differences* (2011): 331-336.

Badr, Hanan E. and Philip M. Moody. "Self-Efficacy: A Predictor for Smoking Cessation Contemplators in Kuwaiti Adults." *International Journal of Behaviorial Medicine* (2005): 273-277.

Barasch, Marc Ian and Caryle Hirshberg. *Remarkable Recovery: What Extraordinary Healings Tell Us About Getting Well and Staying Well.* 1995.

Bar-On, Reuven and James D.A. Parker, *The Handbook of Emotional Intelligence: Theory, Development, Assessment, and applications at Home, School, and in the Workplace.* San Francisco: Jossey-Bass, A Wiley Company, 2000.

Beck, Melinda. "Stress so bad it hurts—Really ." *Wall Street Journal* 17 March 2009: Health Journal.

Boehm, J. K., & Kubzansky, L. D. "The heart's content: The association between positive psychological well-being and cardiovascular health." *Psychological Bulletin* Epub April 2012 (2012): 138(4):655-91 .

Bray, Ilona. *Healthy Employees, Healthy Business.* NOLO, 2009.

Broderick, Jeanine. *Happiness 1st Institute.* n.d.
<http://www.happiness1st.com/index.php/happiness-1st-the-blog/item/your-6th-sense>.

Broderick, Jeanine. "Trusting One's Emotional Guidance Builds Resilience." *Perspectives on Coping and Resilience.* Ed. Venkat Pulla, Shane Warren and Andrew Shatte. Laxmi Nagar: Authors Press, 2013. 254-279.

Brooks, Robert and Sam Goldstein. *The Power of Resilience: Achieving Balance, Confidence, and Personal Strength in Your Life* . McGraw Hill, 2004.

Bruce, Alexandra. *Beyond the Bleep: The definitive unauthorized guide to What the Bleep Do We Know?!* St Paul: Disinformation, 2005.

BTO.org. n.d. 2014. <http://www.bto.org/science/migration/tracking-studies/cuckoo-tracking/what-have-we-learnt>.

BY BRANDEL FRANCE DE BRAVO, MPH, RN SARAH MILLER and AND JESSICA BECKER. *Are E-Cigarettes Safer Than Regular Cigarettes?* n.d. <http://www.stopcancerfund.org/uncategorized/are-e-cigarettes-safer-than-regular-cigarettes/>.

Cancer.gov. n.d. <http://www.cancer.gov/cancertopics/factsheet/Tobacco/smokeless>.

CDC. *Center for Disease Control*. March 2014. 2014. <http://www.cdc.gov/bam/life/frazzled.html>.

Clinic, Mayo. *E-cigarette safety concerns*. n.d. <http://www.mayoclinic.org/healthy-living/quit-smoking/expert-answers/electronic-cigarettes/faq-20057776>.

Conwell, Russell Herman. *Acres of Diamonds: Our everyday opportunities*. Kindle: Public Domain books, 2009.

Danner, DD, DA Snowdon, and WV Friesen. " "Positive Emotions in Early Life and Longevity: Findings from the Nun Study." ." *Journal of Personality and Social Psychology*. (2001): 804-13.

Davis, Amanda. "Seeing with our Brains." 2005. <http://serendip.brynmawr.edu/bb/neuro/neuro05/web2/adavis.html>.

Diener, Ed and Robert Biswas-Diener. *Happiness: Unlocking the Mysteries of Psychological Wealth*. Blackwell Publishing, 2008.

Dockray, Samantha and Andrew Steptoe. "Positive Affect and psychobiological processes." *Neuroscience and Biobehavioral Reviews* (2010): 69-75.

Dukudraw. *5 Blind men and elephant*. Custom drawing--Fiverr. *TRUE Prevention*. Malaysia, 2014.

Ekmund, P. "An argument for basic emotions." *Cognition and Emotion* 6 (1992): 169-200.

Feldman, Barrett L, M. J. Tarr and S. Lebrecht. "'Micro-Valences: Perceiving Affective Valence in Everyday Objects'." *Frontiers in Psychology* (2012).

Ferdinand, keith C., et al. "Health economics of cardiovascular disease: Defining the researchagenda." *CVD Prevention and Control* (2011): 91-100.

Fredrickson, B. L., & Levenson, R. W. "Positive emotions speed recovery from the cardiovascular sequelae of negative emotions." *Cognition and Emotion* (1998): 12: 191-220.

Fredrickson, B. L., and Branigan, C. "Positive Emotions broaden the scope of attention and though-action repertoires." *Cognition and Emotion* (2005): 19: 313-332.

Fredrickson, B. L., Tugade, M. M., et al. "What good are positive emotions in crises?: A Prospective study of resilience and emotions following the terrorist attacks on the United States on September 11, 2001." *Journal of Personality and Social Psychology* (2003): 84: 365-76.

Fredrickson, Barbara L. "The role of positive emotions in positive psychology: The broaden-and-build theory." *American Psychologist* (2001): 56: 218-26.

Fredrickson, Barbara L. *Positivity*. Three Rivers Press, 2010.

Fredrickson, Barbara L. *The Science of Happiness* A. Winter. The Sun Magazine, May 2009.

Frye, Joyce and Barbara Sarter. "Experience With the "Banerji Protocols" in Treatment of Chronic Disease." *Global Advances in Health and Medicine* (2013): 2(Suppl):13B. 4 2014.

Goleman, Daniel. *Social Intelligence*. Bantam Books, 2006.

Gould, Roger L. *Transformations*. New York: Simon and Schuster, 1978.

Gyamfi, Cynthia, Mavis M Gyamfi and Richard L Berkowitz. "Ethical and Medicolegal Considerations in the care of a Jehovah's Witness." *OBSTETRICS & GYNECOLOGY* 1 July 2003.

Haidt, Jonathan. *The Happiness Hypothesis: Finding Modern Truth in Ancient Wisdom*. Basic Books, 2006.

Hanh, Thich Nhat. *Happiness: Essential Mindfulness Practices*. Berkeley: Parallalax, 2009.

Harman, Willis. *Global Mind Change*. Barrett-Koehler Publishers, Inc., 1998.

Holden, Robert. *BE Happy: Release the Power of Happiness in you*. Carlsbad: Hay House, 2009.

—. *Happiness Now: Timeless Wisdom for Feeling Good FAST*. Hay House, 2007.

Hutchins, Max. *Chapter 9: Chemical Senses: Olfaction and Gustation*. n.d. <http://neuroscience.uth.tmc.edu/s2/chapter09.html>.

Ito, T. and G. R. Urland. "Race and gender on the brain: Electro-cortical measures of attention to the race and gender of multiple categorizable individuals." *Journal of Personality and Social Psychology* (2003): 616-26.

Jauch-Chara, Kamilla and Kerstin M. Oltmanns. "Obesity - A neuropsychological disease? Systematic review and neuropsychological model." *Progress in Neurobiology* (2014): xxx-xxx (In Press).

Johnson, K. J., Waugh, C.E., and Fredrickson, B.L. "Smile to see the forest: Facially expressed positive emotions broaden cognition." *COGNITION AND EMOTION* (2010): 24(2): 299-321.

Keller, M. C., Fredrickson, B. L., et al. "A warm heart and a clear head: The contingent effects of mood and weather on cognition." *Psychological Science* (2005): 16: 724-731.

Laitinen, Jaana, Ellen Ek and Ulla Sovio. "Stress Related Eating and Drinking Behavior and BMI and Predictors of this Behavior." *Preventive Medicine* (2002): 29-39.

Lazarus. *Cognition and Emotion.* 1991.

Lewis, Sarah. *Positive Psychology at Wrok: How Positive Leadership and Appreciative Inquiry Create Inspiring Organizations.* Wiley-Blackwell, 2011.

Lipton, Bruch H. and Steve Bhaerman. *Spontaneous Evolution: Our Positive Future (and a way to get there from here).* Carlsbad: Hay House, 2009.

Lloyd, Cathy, Julie Smith and Katie Weinger. "Stress and Diabetes: A Review of the Links." *Diabetes Spectrum* n.d.

Lyubomirsky, Sonja. *The How of Happiness: A Scientific Approach to Getting the Life You Want.* New York: The Penguin Press, 2008.

Martins, Alexandra, Nelson Ramalho and Estelle Morin. "A Comprehensive meta-analysis of the relationship between Emotional Intelligence and health." *Personality and Individual Differences* (2010): 554-564.

McCarthy, Bill and Teresa Casey. "Get Happy! Positive Emotion, Depression and Juvenile Crime." *American Sociological Associaion Annual Meeting.* Las Vegas: UC Davis, 2011.

McClave, Annette K., et al. "Associations between smoking cessation and anxiety and depression." *Addictive Behaviors* (2009): 491-497.

Meissner, C. and J. Brigham. "Thirty yesrs of inevetigating the own-race bias in memory for faces." *Psychology, Public Policy and Law* 7 (2001): 3--35.

Monarch-butterfly.com. n.d. <http://www.monarch-butterfly.com/>.

Nadler, Reldan S. *Leading with emotional Intelligence: Hands-on strategies for building confident and collaborative star performers.* New York: McGraw Hill, 2011.

NIH. *National Institute of Health.* n.d. 2014. <http://www.nlm.nih.gov/medlineplus/magazine/issues/winter08/articles/winter08pg6b.html>.

Nisbett, Richard E. *The Geography of Thought: How Asians and Westerners Think Differently...and Why.* New York: The Free Press, 2003.

Ornstein, Robert E. *The Psychology of Consciousness.* Harcourt Brace Jovanovich, Inc., 1977.

Peil, K.T. "(In press). Emotion: The Self-regulatory Sense." *Global Advances in Health and Medicine* (2012): x(x), xxx-xxx.

Peil, Katherine T. "Emotion: A Self-regulatory Sense." (2014).

Popp, Fritz, et al. "New evidence for Coherence and DNA as Source." *Cell Biophysics* (1984): 33-52.

Pryce-Jones, Jessica. *Happiness at Work: maximizing your Psychological Capital for Success.* Wiley-Blackwell, 2010.

Puhl, Rebecca, Joerg Luedicke and Jamie Lee Peterson. "Public Reactions to Obesity-Related Health Campaigns: A Randomized Controlled Trial." *American Journal of Preventive Medicine* (2013): 45(1): 36-48.

Raedt, Rudi De. "Cognitive Control moderates the association between stress and rumination." *Journal of Behavior Therapy and Experimental Psychiatry* (2012): 519-525.

Rhodes, G. S., Brake and et al. "Expertise and configural coding in race recognition." *British Journal of Psychology* (1989): 313-31.

Ricard, Matthieu. *Happiness: A Guide to Developing Life's Most Important Skill.* Little, Brown and Company, 2003.

Roger VL, Go AS, Lloyd-Jones DM, Benjamin EJ, Berry JD, Borden WB, Bravata DM, Dai S, Ford ES, Fox CS, Fullerton HJ, Gillespie C, Hailpern SM, Heit JA, Howard VJ, Kissela BM, Kittner SJ, Lackland DT, Lichtman JH, Lisabeth LD, Makuc DM, Marcus GM, Marelli. "Heart disease and stroke statistics--2012 update: a report from the American Heart Association." n.d.

Rubenstein, Ed. *An Awakening from the Trances of Everyday Life: A Journey to Empowerment.* Sages Way Press, 1999.

Salwen, J. K. et al. "Childhood abuse, adult interpersonal abuse, and depression in individuals with extreme obesity." *Child Abuse & Neglect* (2014). <http://dx.doi.org/10.1016/j.chiabu.2013.12.005>.

Sarno, John. *Healing Back Pain: The Mind-Body Connection.* New York: Warner, 1991.

Sbarra, , D. A., H. L. Smith and M. R. Mehl. "Advice to divorcees: Go easy on yourself." *Association for Psychological Science* (2001).

Schneider, Tamera R. "The role of neuroticism on psychological and physiological stress responses." *Journal of Experimental Social Psychology* (2004): 795-804.

Schwarz, David J. *The Magic of Thinking BIG.* New York: Simon & Schuster, 1959 (2007).

Seligman, M. E. P. *Flourish: A Visionary New Understanding of Happiness and Well-Being.* New York: Free Press, 2011.

Seligman, M.E.P., Noeln-Hoekosema, S., Thornton, N. & Thornton, K.M. "Explanatory style as a mechanism of disappointing athletic performance." *Psychological Science* (1990): 1:143-146.

Seligman, Martin E. P. *Authentic Happiness: Using the new positive psychology to realize your potential for lasting fulfillment.* New York: Free Press, 2002.

Seligman,, Martin E. P. Ph.D. *Learned Optimism.* Originally published 1991. New York: Simon & Schuster, 2006.

Shahar, Tal Ben. *Happier*. New York: McGraw Hill, 2007.

Shapiro, Marcey. *Transforming the Nature of Health: A Holistic Vision of Healthing That Honors Our Connection to the Earth, Others, and Ourselves*. Berkeley: North Atlantic Books, 2012.

Shenk, David. *The Genius in All of Us*. Doubleday, 2010.

Siebert, Al. *The Resiliency Advantage: Master Change, Thrive under Pressure, and Bounce Back from Setbacks*. San Francisco: Berrett-Koehler Publishers, Inc., 2005.

Siebold, Steve. *177 Mental Toughness Secrets of the World Class*. London House, 2010.

Simonton, O Carl, Stephanie Simonton and James L Creighton. *Getting well again : a step-by-step, self-help guide to overcoming cancer for patients and their families*. New York: St Martin's Press, 1978.

Talbot, Michael. *The Holographic Universe*. New York: Harper Collins, 1991.

Thurston, Rebecca C., Marissa Rewak and Laura D. Kubzansky. "An Anxious Heart: Anxiety and the Onset of Cardiovascular Diseases." *Progress in Cardiovascular Diseases* (2013): 524-537.

Tugade, M. M., and Fredrickson, B. L. "Resilient Individuals use positive emotions to bounce back from negative emotional experiences." *Journal of Personality and Social Psychology* (2004): Journal of Personaltiy and Social Psychology.

Virginia Hill Rice, Ph.D., RN. " Theories of Stress and its Relationship to Health." *Handbook of Stress, Coping, and Health, Implications for Nursing Research, Theory, and Practice*. Second Edition . Save Publication, Inc., 2012. Chapter 2.

Waugh, C. E., Fredrickson, B. L., and Taylor, S. F. "Adapting to life's slings and arrows: Individual differences in resilience when recovering from an unanticipated threat." *Journal of Research in Personality* (2008): 42: 1031-46.

WHO. n.d. <http://www.who.int/mediacentre/factsheets/fs317/en/>.

Wilkinson, Kirk. *The Happiness Factor: How to be Happy No Matter What!* Austin: Ovation Books, 2008.

Winseman, Albert L., Donald O. Clifton and Curt Liesveld. *Living Your Strengths*. New York: Gallup Press, 2003.

Wittayanukorn, Saranrat, Jingjing Qian and Richard A. Hansen. "Prevalence of depressive symptoms and predictors of treatment among US adults from 2005 to 2010." *General Hospital Psychiatry* (2014): xxx-xxx (In Press).

Zhuo, Xiaohui, Ping Zhang and Thomas J. Hoerger. "Lifetime Direct Medical Costs of Treating Type 2 Diabetes and Diabetic Complications." *American journal of Preventive Medicine* (2013): 253-261.

[1] (Gyamfi, Gyamfi and Berkowitz)
[2] (Lyubomirsky)

[4] (WHO)
[5] **2,717,991 retrieved from** (143)
[6] (Roger VL)
[7] (Boehm)
[8] (Ferdinand, Orenstein and Hong)
[99] (Ferdinand, Orenstein and Hong)
[10] (Boehm)
[11] (Danner)
[12] (Puhl, Luedicke and Peterson)
[13] (Lewis)
[14] (McClave, Dube and Strine)
[15] (McClave, Dube and Strine)
[16] (McClave, Dube and Strine)
[17] (Covey, Glassman, & Stetner, 1998)
[18] (Covey et al, 2003)
[19] (Badr and Moody)
[20] (McClave, Dube and Strine)
[21] (McClave, Dube and Strine)
[22] The man referenced has long since passed away.
[23] (BY BRANDEL FRANCE DE BRAVO, SARAH MILLER and BECKER) (Cancer.gov)
[24] (Clinic)
[25] (Puhl, Luedicke and Peterson)
[26] (Laitinen, Ek and Sovio) (Andrews, Lowe and Clair)
[27] (Jauch-Chara and Oltmanns)
[28] (Puhl, Luedicke and Peterson)
[29] (Salwen)
[30] (Wittayanukorn, Qian and Hansen)
[31] (Dockray and Steptoe)
[32] Note to researchers: The same argument holds true if the depression caused by unmanaged stress is only 50%. As long as we study such cases with those whose roots may be caused by other factors, our sample is diluted and solutions are delayed.
[33] (Bray)
[34] (Thurston, Rewak and Kubzansky)
[35] (Raedt)
[36] (Lloyd, Smith and Weinger)
[37] (Zhuo, Zhang and Hoerger)
[38] (Zhuo, Zhang and Hoerger)
[39] (Sarno)
[40] (Beck)
[41] (Armstrong, Galligan and Critchley)
[42] (M. E. Seligman)
[43] (B. L. Fredrickson, The Science of Happiness)

[44] (K. T. Peil)
[45] (UCARC)
[46] (B. L. Fredrickson, Positivity)
[47] (B. L. Fredrickson, The Science of Happiness)
[48] (Ong, Bergeman, Bisconti & Wallace, 2006)
[49] I'm not sure what to call this, perhaps sense of taste. Although I was taught that taste buds are on the tongue, more recent research has demonstrated that taste is a combination of senses, some in the nasal passages, some on the tongue, and some in the intestines, which are combined with other things before our conscious brain recognizes the taste of something.
[50] (Hutchins)
[51] (Davis)
[52] (BTO.org)
[53] (Monarch-butterfly.com)
[54] (BTO.org)
[55] (Harman)
[56] (Frye and Sarter)
[57] (Goldstein)
[58] (Goldstein)
[59] (Lebrecht, Bar, Feldman, Barrett, & Tarr, 2012)
[60] (Ricard)
[61] (Schneider)
[62] (Lewis)
[63] Unpublished manuscript (Shades of Joy)
[64] (Simonton, Simonton and Creighton)
[65] This link was referenced in another report citing (Matthews and Glass, 1981). I have been unable to find this research despite several hours of searching. If anyone has access to it, or information about it, I would be most appreciative of receiving an update.
[66] (Barasch and Hirshberg)
[67] (Virginia Hill Rice)
[68] The EGS is a compilation of similar scales used by a variety of teachers including David Hawkins, L. Ron Hubbard, and Abraham Hicks. The zones are my addition. The science supporting the emotional guidance scale, or that emotions provide guidance, did not exist when the earlier scales were created. I have applied the science explaining the scale to their earlier work and found the Hicks scale most closely matches current science. All emotions could be placed on the scale. It is simplified to reflect emotions that are similar in degrees of empowerment in each zone.
[69] (K. T. Peil)
[70] (Peil)
[71] (Peil)
[72] (B. L. Fredrickson)

[73] (Lazarus)
[74] (B. L. Fredrickson)
[75] There is a plethora of growing evidence suggesting that social ills (crime, teen pregnancy, drug and alcohol abuse, and more) are casually related to long-term emotional pain. There is also mounting evidence that links improved desirable behaviors are increased through positive emotion including better corporate citizenship, altruism, kindness to strangers without expectation of reward, better relationships of all types, and much more. (Pryce-Jones) (B. L. Fredrickson, Positivity) (McCarthy and Casey)
[76] (M. Seligman)
[77] (Rubenstein)
[78] (B. L. Fredrickson, Positivity)
[79] (Ekmund)
[80] (Rubenstein)
[81] (Talbot)
[82] (Ricard)
[83] (Oregon State University , 2012)
[84] (Montgomery, 2012)
[85] (Feldman, Tarr and Lebrecht)
[86] (Sbarra, , Smith and Mehl)
[87] (B. L. Fredrickson) (B. L. Fredrickson, The Science of Happiness) (Seligman,) (M. Seligman) (Achor)
[88] (Peil, 2012)
[89] (Seligman, 2006)
[90] (Brooks and Goldstein)
[91] (M. Seligman)
[92] (Brooks and Goldstein)
[93] (Brooks, Goldstein 2004)
[94] (Rubenstein) (Brooks and Goldstein)
[95] (Brooks and Goldstein)
[96][96] (Brooks, Goldstein 2004)
[97] (Brooks, Goldstein 2004)
[98] (M. N.-H. Seligman)
[99] (Brooks, Goldstein 2004)
[100] (Brooks, Goldstein 2004)

Bibliography

[101] (Rubenstein)
[102] (Nisbett)
[103] (Ornstein)
[104] (Haidt)
[105] (Lipton and Bhaerman)
[106] (Peil)
[107] (Ito and Urland) (Johnson) (Meissner and Brigham)
[108] (Schwarz)
[109] (Diener and Biswas-Diener)
[110] (Rollin & Atkinson, 2004)
[111] (Nadler)
[112] (Bruce)
[113] (Goleman)
[114] Because of all the benefits of positivity (kinder, healthier, increased cognitive ability, etc.)
[115] (Popp, Nagl and Wolf)
[116] Although research has reported this link, they have not been able to explain it. I believe the answer will be found in the connections we form on the quantum level.
[117] (Bandura)
[118] (CDC)
[119] (NIH)
[120] (Boehm)
[121] (Broderick, Happiness 1st Institute)
[122] (GradDipClinNsg, Wilkes BSc PhD RN CM MHPEd GradDipEd(Nur and Luke RN BN DipNsg)
[123] (Wilkinson)
[124] (Winseman, Clifton and Liesveld)
[125] See: Emotion: A Self-Regulatory Sense (www.emotionalsentience.com) by K. T. Peil, Harvard, 2012
[126] (Hanh)
[127] I've seen this increase income in < 1 year by 60%. It has to do with both expectation and belief in our self and worthiness.
[128] (Shenk)
[129] (Siebert)
[130] (B. L. Fredrickson) studies
[131] (Holden)
[132] (Shapiro)
[133] (Shahar)